Thaís Braga de Paula

Sodium in French bread from supermarket bakeries in Brazil

Thaís Braga de Paula

Sodium in French bread from supermarket bakeries in Brazil

Analytical observational cross-sectional study

ScienciaScripts

Cover image: www.ingimage.com

This book is a translation from the original published under ISBN 978-613-9-68685-8.

Publisher:
Sciencia Scripts
is a trademark of
Dodo Books Indian Ocean Ltd. and OmniScriptum S.R.L publishing group

120 High Road, East Finchley, London, N2 9ED, United Kingdom
Str. Armeneasca 28/1, office 1, Chisinau MD-2012, Republic of Moldova, Europe
Printed at: see last page
ISBN: 978-620-8-22716-6

CONTENTS

SUMMARY

High salt intake is one of the main risk factors for cardiovascular disease. Considering bread as a food widely consumed by the Brazilian population, the aim of this study was to analyze the sodium content and production method of French bread made in supermarket bakeries in Goiânia-GO, with a view to assessing compliance with the voluntary sodium reduction agreement. This is an analytical observational cross-sectional study carried out in 23 medium and large supermarkets selected by random drawing. Two samples were taken from four units of French bread and the sodium content was analyzed by diluting the ash in acid and reading it in a flame photometer. A questionnaire was administered at the sites visited on aspects related to production. The sodium content ranged from 286 to 702 mg/100g of bread. Only two supermarkets had bread samples above 586 mg/100g, the maximum reference value. Of the samples analyzed, 82.6% weighed more than 50g per unit. In the bivariate analysis, supermarkets that use their own recipe produce bread with a lower sodium content than those that use premix. Those that reduced the salt in the recipe had bread with a lower sodium content. No association was found between the sodium content of the bread and the use of scales, technical data sheets or training for employees. The voluntary agreement was complied with in 91.3% of the sites studied. However, as 78% of the sites reported that they had not changed their recipe after signing the agreement, they could already be producing low-content bread. In addition, the bread units weighed more than the recommended one portion, leading to a higher than expected sodium intake.

Key words: dietary sodium chloride, salt, bread, food production.

CHAPTER 1

1 INTRODUCTION

Changes in the dietary profile of the world's population, characterized by an increase in the consumption of food away from home and processed foods, pose major challenges for public policies, particularly in the area of chronic non-communicable diseases (NCDs) (BROWN et al., 2009).

The National Food and Nutrition Policy (PNAN), the Food Guide for the Brazilian Population and the World Health Organization (WHO) guide the moderate use of added salt, as well as limiting the use of ready-to-eat food products, claiming that these products tend to be nutritionally unbalanced and can lead to great damage to health (MINISTÉRIO DA SAÙDE, 2012; MYSTERY OF HEALTH, 2014; WHO, 2004).

With the aim of promoting the development and implementation of effective and sustainable public policies for the prevention and control of NCDs and risk factors, the Ministry of Health has launched the "Strategic Action Plan for Tackling NCDs in Brazil from 2011 to 2022". Among the national targets proposed for healthier eating and the prevention of CNCDs in this plan is a reduction in the average consumption of salt by the population, based on agreements with the food industry with the aim of reducing the salt content in their products and improving access to less salty processed foods (MINISTERIO DA SAUDE, 2011a).

One of the main strategies used to reduce salt consumption in food reformulation has been the gradual reduction of this ingredient in processed products. This strategy has been evaluated as an advantageous method, considering that the perception of the sensory attributes of the foods involved does not seem to change, since consumers' taste buds adjust over time to the lower level of salt (LIEM; MIREMADI; KEAST, 2011; MCLEAN, 2014). This mechanism of taste adaptation has not yet been fully elucidated (which biochemical/sensory mechanism is involved, how long adaptation takes, interferences in the process, etc.), but it is known that the perception and preference of salty tastes are more closely linked to individual habits in relation to the regular consumption of salt in the concentrations to which they are accustomed (BANNWART; SILVA; VIDAL, 2014). It is also worth noting that repeated exposure to low-sodium diets results in greater sensitivity to salty tastes (COBCROFT; TIKELLIS; BUSCH, 2008).

In order to propose a gradual reduction in the salt content of bread, the Ministry of Health, the Brazilian Association of Food Industries (ABIA), the Brazilian Association of Pasta Industries (ABIMA), the Brazilian Wheat Industry Association (ABITRIGO) and the Brazilian Bakery and Confectionery Industry Association (ABIP) signed a Commitment Agreement in 2011 to reduce the salt content in various products, including French bread, by the end of 2014 (MINISTÉRIO DA SAÙDE, 2011b).

In Brazil, data from the last Household Budget Survey (POF), which took place between 2008 and 2009, showed that Brazilians consume approximately 53 g of French bread a day, which is equivalent to one unit a day (IBGE, 2010). Considering the sodium content of French bread is 324 mg/50 g (NEPA, 2011), the consumption of one unit of French bread per day corresponds to 16% of the recommended daily sodium requirement (2000 mg) (WHO, 2012).

Thus, based on the standard French bread formulation, which in 2011 contained 2 g of salt/100 g of wheat flour, the National Health Surveillance Agency (ANVISA) proposed a reduction to 1.8 g of salt/100 g of wheat flour, i.e. a 10% reduction in salt. The proposal was to gradually reduce the sodium content to a maximum of 586 mg of sodium/100 g of French bread by 2014 (MINISTÉRIO DA SAÙDE, 2011b). With this reduction, the consumption of one unit of French bread (50 g) would correspond to 14.65% of the daily sodium requirement.

Although scientific evidence from the results observed in developed countries indicates that salt reduction policies focused on processed foods may be feasible at the population level, data on the effectiveness and impact of these interventions remain limited in developing countries, such as Brazil (FERRANTE et al., 2011). This highlights the need for more studies to monitor the policies developed in the country and compliance with voluntary agreements and their effectiveness, in order to guarantee a real reduction in salt and sodium in processed foods with an effect on the health of the population.

In view of the above, this study was motivated by: the importance of the continued contribution of scientific research into sodium consumption, in terms of public health and for the food industry; the scarcity of studies that monitor the policies that have been developed in Brazil, the evaluation of compliance with voluntary agreements and knowledge about how French bread is produced in relation to sodium content in order to support and assist new and successive reductions with a view to reducing the prevalence of chronic non-communicable diseases in the population.

2 LITERATURE REVIEW

2.1 GENERAL AND HISTORICAL ASPECTS

Sodium chloride (NaCl), better known as "table salt", is currently considered the main source of sodium in Western diets and contributes around 90% of the total intake of this nutrient. In a salt crystal, the mass ratio is 60% chloride and 40% sodium (BANNWART; SILVA; VIDAL, 2014).

In nature, there are two types of salt: "sea salt", which is obtained by evaporating sea water, and "rock salt", which is extracted from underground rocks resulting from lakes and seas that have dried up. However, the market sells various types of salt, such as refined salt and coarse salt (400 mg of sodium / 1 g of salt), dietary salt or light salt, which has 50% sodium chloride and 50% potassium chloride (200 mg of sodium / 1 g of salt), fleur de sel (small crystals formed on the surfaces of salt pans by the action of the wind) and salts that are named after the region in which they are extracted, often rock salts, such as Peruvian pink salt, Himalayan pink salt, Hawaiian salt, among others. It's worth noting that what sets these salts apart is precisely the fact that they are unrefined, which gives them the presence (in small quantities, but more than refined salt) of other minerals such as magnesium, calcium, iron and potassium. The amount of sodium is usually similar to refined table salt (DRAKE; DRAKE, 2011).

Historically, salt has always had a symbolic value associated with its image, giving it socio-cultural and economic importance. Economically, it was used as a form of payment for soldiers in Ancient Rome, from where the name salàrio later arose. In terms of cultural importance, the prefix "salt" has been incorporated into the names of some European cities (Salzburg in Austria, Saltcotes in Scotland, Salzkotten and Salzuflen in Germany, among others) (RITZ, 1996).

It is also worth adding that some historical records in European countries mention the intake of quite high levels of salt. In Sweden in the 16th century, the reported daily intake was 100g of salt, mainly due to the diet based on cured foods. In Denmark, on the other hand, an intake of 50 g/day was observed. However, in countries such as 17th century France, where heavy taxes were imposed on salt, consumption was lower, at 13 to 15 g/day (RITZ, 1996). In addition, the arrival of refrigerators allowed the population to abandon salting methods, reducing the amount of salt ingested.

The World Health Organization (WHO) recommends a daily intake of no more than 5 g of salt (2000 mg of sodium) for adults (WHO, 2012). In recent decades, salt consumption in most countries has been excessive, ranging from 9 to 12 g per person per day (BROWN et al., 2009).

Cordain et al. (2005) analyzed the Western diet and its origins and found that the proportion of sodium and potassium intake has radically reversed when compared to the Paleolithic diet (essential consumption of meat and vegetables), due to the increase in consumption of salty and processed foods and the decrease in fruit and vegetable intake. This disproportion between sodium and potassium is considered harmful and can lead to chronic non-communicable diseases.

Studies also point to the positive correlation between sodium intake and some diseases such as gastric cancer (TSUGANE et al., 2004), hypertension and cardiovascular diseases (MENETON et al., 2005), kidney stones (OBLIGADO; GOLDFARB, 2008), diabetes, osteoporosis, reduced bone density, alongside other factors such as obesity, smoking and a sedentary lifestyle (BROWN et al., 2009; HE; MACGREGOR, 2009).

The mechanisms by which sodium affects blood pressure (BP) have not yet been fully elucidated (BANNWART; SILVA; VIDAL, 2014).). The response to high salt intake differs between salt-sensitive and non-salt-sensitive individuals. It is suggested that individuals who are more sensitive to salt, when consuming too much, will not excrete sodium properly, which promotes the expansion of plasma volume, which in turn increases intracellular volume, causing an increase in peripheral resistance and extracellular volume, with a consequent increase in blood pressure. In non-salt sensitive individuals, excretion is adapted to intake (POTTER; PERRY, 2005; SCHMIDLIN et al., 2007). A universal definition of salt sensitivity should be better explored in longitudinal studies (TAVARES; JUNIOR KOHLMANN, 2004).

However, the scientific evidence regarding sodium intake and BP elevation has been pointed out as one of the strongest cause and effect relationships among all the existing dietary factors associated with the onset of cardiovascular diseases, which justifies global initiatives to reduce consumption of this nutrient (KOTCHEN, COWLEY, FROHLIC, 2013; WHO, 2007).

2.2 FUNCTIONS OF SODIUM IN THE HUMAN BODY AND SALT IN FOOD AND BAKED GOODS

Although scientific evidence points to the need to reduce sodium in the diet, it should also be considered that sodium performs important functions in the body. These include the osmotic regulation of fluids, the transmission of nerve impulses, muscle action, helping glands to function and maintaining acid-base balance (STRAZZULLO; LECLERCQ, 2014).

For the body to function properly, it is estimated that the minimum physiological need for sodium is around 200 to 500 mg/day (WHO, 2012). A healthy adult has around 90 g of sodium in the body, of which 50% is in the extracellular fluid and the rest in the intracellular fluid and bones (STRAZZULLO; LECLERCQ, 2014).

In addition to its health functions, salt also plays many roles in food. There are reports that the use of salt to preserve perishable foods began around 5,000 years ago with the Chinese. This processing facilitated the phenomenon of sedentarization of the human race, which from then on could store the food collected and hunted one day and consume it at another time (BANNWART; SILVA; VIDAL, 2014).

Salt, especially sodium, is the element that best promotes the salty taste that is part of the five basic tastes perceived by humans. The salty taste basically comes from the interaction between some metallic ions, which could be sodium, lithium and potassium, with receptors on the tongue's epithelial cells. Lithium is toxic when ingested in medium quantities and other ions, such as potassium, have a metallic taste associated with a salty taste (CHANDRASHEKAR et al., 2010). In addition, sodium salts can also influence the overall taste of food by enhancing the most present flavor, be it bitter, sour or sweet (BRESLIN; SPECTOR, 2008).

It is also worth noting that the addition of salt promotes effects on the processed food, such as longer shelf life, better flavor and texture. At the same time, it is one of the lowest-cost additives in formulations. In preservation, it acts by retaining water in foods with a high moisture content and has an inhibiting effect on the growth of microorganisms in the food (HUTTON, 2002; MAN, 2007).

In terms of texture, it is particularly useful in the bakery industry, as it firms up the gluten network and makes it more stable and less extensible. It also helps with the fermentation process, because the more salt you add to the dough, the longer the yeast has to act. With this longer time, more gases are released, thus increasing the expansion of the bread with a consequent effect on the texture, making it softer (HUTTON, 2002).

It is worth considering that the absence of salt affects the growth of bread, as a weaker gluten network is formed, as well as reducing the overall quality of the bread, producing a less crunchy crust, a less salty taste and a shorter shelf life for the product. On the other hand, excess salt also impairs the fermentation of baked goods by inhibiting the development of yeast (ANVISA, 2012a). However, the salt content for one or the other is not reported in the literature.

Promoting these effects in food without considering the health factor can contribute to the high sodium content in food produced by industries. Examples of processed foods with a high sodium content include various types of cheese, canned foods, most sausages, ready-made seasonings and concentrates, among others, with average levels (mg /100 g) ranging from 926, 1,567, 1,039 and 32,560, respectively (LIEM; MIREMADI; KEAST, 2011;

NEPA, 2011).

2.3 CONSUMPTION AND REDUCTION OF SODIUM CONTENT IN FOODS

Sodium consumption by the world's population is well above the latest recommendation from the World Health Organization in 2012 (WHO, 2012). It is recommended that intake should not exceed 2000 mg of sodium or 5 grams of salt per day. In many countries, the recommended maximum daily intake of sodium is 2300 mg/day (USDA, 2010). Brazilian labeling uses the recommended daily value of 2400 mg/day for a 2000 Kcal diet (BRASIL, 2003). However, there is evidence to suggest that sodium intake should be even lower, from 1200 to 1500 mg/day, when considering its impact on health (DOTSH et al., 2009).

As human society has been organized in a multicultural way, there is great variability in the amount of salt ingested by different populations. Page, Damon and Moellering (1974) reported on the salt consumption of six tribes in the Solomon Islands, a small country in the Pacific, and all the tribesmen, who were faithful to their culture, had a higher sodium intake when compared to those who had had contact with Western culture.

The societies with the lowest levels of sodium intake were the Yanomami and Xingu tribes of Brazil and the rural populations of Kenya, who ingested around 0.4-1.2 mg/day, or 1-3 g/day of salt (TEKOL, 2006).

The data in Table 1 shows the average values of salt and sodium intake in the adult population of some countries in studies published in the last 10 years (2007 to 2017).

Table 1. Salt and sodium consumption in the adult population of some countries.

Parents	**Amount of salt ingested (g/day)**	**Amount of sodium ingested (mg/day)**
Chile (VALENZUELA et al., 2014)	12,00	4.800
Brazil (SARNO et al., 2013)	11,75	4.700
Denmark (ANDERSEN et al., 2009)	10,00	4.000
Wales (NATIONAL CENTRE FOR SOCIAL RESEARCH, 2007)	8,60	3.440
Canada (CAMPBELL; JOHNSON; CAMPBELL, 2011)	8,50	3.400
USA (PFEIFFER et al., 2014)	8,50	3.400

South Africa (BERTRAM et al., 2012)	8,10	3.240
WHO recommendation (WHO, 2012)	**5**	**2.000**

Countries such as Canada, the USA, Wales and South Africa had similar intakes of salt and sodium per day, at around 1.7 times the WHO recommendation. Denmark, Brazil and Chile, on the other hand, consumed more than twice the recommended amount. This data confirms the worldwide concern about excessive sodium consumption.

Taking into account the sources of sodium in the diet, in the population of European countries and the United States (USA), sodium consumption comes mainly, from 75 to 90%, from processed foods and/or foods served in restaurants. In Asian countries, a large part of sodium consumption comes from the addition of salt in food preparation, the use of soy sauce, miso (a preparation typical of Japanese culture) and foods in brine (BROWN et al., 2009).

In Brazil, data from the latest study on salt and sodium consumption at a population level shows a different profile from other countries. Data from the POF 2008-2009 showed that almost 75% of the salt ingested in Brazil comes from added salt or processed seasonings with added sodium chloride. Natural foods, or those without added sodium, only account for 4.8% of total intake. Processed foods have increased their contribution to individuals' sodium intake by 18.9% (SARNO et al., 2013).

More recent studies such as VIGITEL in 2014, when estimating the impact of a high-sodium diet, found that only 15.5% of the people interviewed recognized the high or very high salt content of food (VIGITEL, 2014). Consumers are often unaware of the amount of salt present in the processed foods they eat regularly. A classic example is French bread, which contains around 648 mg of sodium/100 g (NEPPA, 2011). As the population is not aware of the concentration of salt present, because it is not easily perceived by taste, if you consume more than one portion a day you could be ingesting a high sodium content (NWANGUMA; OKORIE, 2013).

In addition, the amount of each food consumed is also a factor that influences total daily sodium intake. Bread and cookies do not normally have a high sodium content in one portion, but they are consumed in many portions and can contribute 35 to 50% of the daily sodium intake (COTTON et al., 2004).

Some studies have been carried out on breads with a lower sodium content and consumer acceptance has been verified. La Croix et al. (2015) reported that the 10% sodium reduction in breads made with 50% whole wheat flour was not perceived by consumers, and the 30% sodium reduction, although detected, did not bring any negative aspects to the evaluation. Girgis et al. (2003) showed that the progressive and gradual reduction of the sodium content in white bread by up to 25% over six weeks had no influence on the acceptability to consumers. Bolhuis et al. (2011) managed to reduce the sodium content by 52% in wholemeal bread with various sandwich fillings without altering consumer acceptability.

A study carried out in the United Kingdom found more than 1200 mg of sodium/100 g of the bread analyzed (equivalent to 3 g of salt in two pieces of bread), which shows how significant this food is in terms of the amount of sodium ingested (MHURCHU et al., 2011). Another study carried out in this country showed that the sodium content has been progressively reduced, but that there is still great variation between the different types of bread, which indicates that further reductions could be made (BRINSDEN et al., 2013). In this sense, the United Kingdom has been a world leader in reducing sodium in food.

Also in this context, some groups have carried out research into average sodium intake in various societies and social groups. These include INTERSALT and INTERMAP. INTERSALT was a standardized epidemiological study on a worldwide scale (32 countries) involving 10,079 men and women between the ages of 20 and 59, which tested the correlation between sodium intake, analyzed by its excretion in the urine over 24 hours, and blood pressure. The results proved the hypothesis, as well as other studies (COOK, et al., 2007; GELEIJNSE; KOK; GROBBEE, 2003; HE; MACGREGOR, 2002), that excess salt intake is strongly linked to the development of cardiovascular diseases (ELLIOTT et al., 1996; STAMLER, 1997).

INTERMAP, on the other hand, was an epidemiological study that aimed to establish relationships between dietary factors and cardiovascular diseases in the various countries studied (China, the United States, Japan and the United Kingdom). However, what set it apart from other studies in the field was that it analyzed dietary factors that had not yet been explored, such as the quantity and quality of protein, amino acids, lipids and carbohydrates ingested, as well as the influence of various ions on the development of heart disease. Finally, this study verified the relationship between the factors studied and cardiovascular diseases according to the level of education of the consumers. People with a lower level of education showed greater adverse effects on blood pressure, due to higher body mass indexes and other diet-related factors (STAMLER et al., 2003a; STAMLER et al., 2003b).

2.3.1 Sodium reduction programs

Programs for the gradual reduction of sodium have been established by public bodies and authorities, in conjunction with the food industry and opinion formers, in various countries, in various food categories. In 2011, 32 programs to reduce sodium consumption were identified around the world, nineteen of them in Europe, seven in Asia and Oceania, six in the Americas and one in Africa. Examples include Italy (*Gaining Health*), Belgium (*Federal Nutrition Plan for Nutrition & Health*), Sweden, Denmark and Poland (*National Strategy for Sodium Reduction*), Hungary (*Hungarian Salt Reduction Program),* Canada (*Health Canada Multi Stakeholder Working Group on Sodium Reduction*), Turkey and South Africa (*Use Salt Sparingly*) (BANNWART; SILVA; VIDAL,

2014; BARR, 2010). Among the 32 participants, five countries demonstrated the effectiveness of their projects: Finland, France, Ireland, Japan and the United Kingdom (WEBSTER et al., 2011).

In the UK, the *Food Standards Agency* (FSA) has set salt reduction targets for 80 food categories. According to the government, an analysis of progress and targets is carried out every two years and this nutrition policy work has recently become the responsibility of the UK Department of Health (MHURCHU et al., 2011).

In Brazil, the process of setting targets takes into account elements inspired by international experiences, such as those in the United Kingdom and Canada, along with aspects and innovations from the recent Brazilian experience. In 2010, the Brazilian government launched campaigns to reduce sodium consumption in various sectors through the Ministry of Health, based on the "Strategic Action Plan to Combat NCDs in Brazil 2011 - 2022" (MINISTÉRIO DA SAÙDE, 2011a).

Strategies to reduce sodium consumption in the country have as their pillars the promotion of healthy eating, educational actions supported and/or promoted by the government for health professionals, food manufacturers and the general population, as well as the reformulation of processed foods (NILSON; JAIME; RESENDE, 2012).

A voluntary agreement called the "Plan for the Reduction of Sodium in Processed Foods", which is part of the "Plan for the Reduction of Salt Consumption by the Brazilian Population", was signed by the food industries and the Ministry of Health, with the aim of gradually and sustainably reducing the maximum sodium content in different food categories by 2020. For priority food categories, the maximum sodium content limits have already been set, such as bread, broths and seasonings, sausages and mayonnaise, while for others these limits are still being discussed. It is worth adding that the foods were chosen based on the contribution of these categories to the population's sodium intake, associating the total consumption of the product and the average sodium content present in the food (NILSON; JAIME; RESENDE, 2012).

The axes for monitoring these actions are the survey of food nutrition labeling, the survey of the evolution of the use of the main ingredients containing sodium (salt and additives) by food industries and laboratory analysis of food, carried out by the official laboratories of each state or those located closest (MINISTÉRIO DA SAÙDE, 2011b).

Table 2 shows the average sodium content of the foods analyzed as part of the Food Sodium Monitoring Program on a continuous basis. Various brands consumed by the Brazilian population were analyzed. The data presented below refer to the last five technical reports published on research carried out between 2009 and 2015, according to Technical Reports No. 43/2010 (ANVISA, 2010), No. 50/2012 (ANVISA, 2012b), No. 54/2013 (ANVISA, 2013), No. 61/2014 (ANVISA, 2014) and No. 69/2015 (ANVISA, 2015).

Table 2. Average values of the sodium content of foods studied in 2011 and 2012, continuously by the Food Sodium Monitoring Program.

Product Analyzed	**Average sodium content found (mg/ 100g)**		**Highest sodium content found (mg/ 100g)**		**Lowest sodium content found (mg/ 100g)**		**Relationship Major/minor**	
	2011	2012	2011	2012	2011	2012	2011	2012
Straw potatoes	472	205	719	430	250	30	2,9	14,3
Cookie sprinkles	1.092	1.517	1.398	1.988	427		3,3	2
Macaroni instant	1.798	1.881	2.160	2.385	1.435	1.582	1,5	1,5
Cheese bread	558	534	830	747	105	264	7,9	2,8
Frozen cheese bread	582	560	782	648	367	478	2,1	1,3

Minas frescal cheese	505	400	1.819	533	126	264	14,4	2
Mozzarella cheese	577	594	1.068	1.140	309	250	3,5	4,6
Cheese	1402	766	3.052	1.130	223	533	13,7	2,1
parmesan	571	657	986	1.450	326	430	3	3,4
Dish cheese								
Low-calorie soft drinks	12	10	17	19	7	3	2,4	6,3
Corn snacks	779	715	1395	1.415	395	372	3,5	3,8

Source: ANVISA (2011; 2012b)

In the analysis of the evolution of sodium in some foods, instant noodles and cookies had the highest sodium concentrations in the studies carried out in 2011 and 2012 and had a higher sodium content in 2012 compared to the previous year. Also noteworthy was parmesan cheese, which had high concentrations in 2011 but decreased in 2012. In addition, potato sticks had a high increase in sodium content rather than a reduction, followed by low-calorie guarana soft drinks, mozzarella cheese, prato cheese and corn snacks. The other foods either decreased or remained at similar levels.

In 2014, technical report no. 61/2014 published analyses of just three types of food: instant noodles, bread rolls and biscuits. With regard to instant noodles, there was a higher maximum value (2,813 mg of sodium/100 g) and a much lower minimum value (666 mg of sodium/100 g) than in the two previous reports, but in relation to the average of all the samples, the value was not very different. Bread obtained higher average, minimum and maximum values than in the previous studies. There are no previous references for bisnaguinha bread (ANVISA, 2014).

In 2015, monitoring of the sodium content of products that are part of the second agreement signed was launched, including French bread. The results of these analyses included 39 products from 19 different states, including

Goiás. The average sodium content found was 736 mg/100g, with results ranging from 411 mg to 880 mg. The difference between the products with the highest and lowest values was 2.1 times. In addition, as the analyses for this monitoring were carried out in 2014, the sodium values forecast for the end of 2012, which were 616 mg/100g of bread, were used as targets. Thus, in relation to the average (736 mg/100g), the products did not meet the target and only five brands had values lower than the maximum, although the states to which they belonged were not mentioned (ANVISA, 2015). To date, no new monitoring has been launched.

3 OBJECTIVES

3.1 GENERAL OBJECTIVE

To analyze the sodium content and learn about the production method of French bread produced in supermarket bakeries in the municipality of Goiânia-Goiâs, Brazil.

3.2 SPECIFIC OBJECTIVES

✓ To analyze the weight of French bread produced in the bakeries of the supermarkets studied.

✓ Analyze the moisture and sodium content of the bread.

✓ Analyze the sodium content of premixes sold/used in the municipality for making French bread.

✓ Evaluate compliance with the Term of Commitment signed by various food/bakery industry associations and the Ministry of Health.

✓ To analyze the production method of French bread associated with the sodium content of the bakeries studied.

4 MATERIAL AND METHODS

4.1 TYPE AND PLACE OF STUDY

This is an analytical observational cross-sectional study carried out in the municipality of Goiânia-Goiàs, Brazil.

4.2 POPULATION AND SAMPLING

In 2015, there were 344 regularized supermarkets in Goiânia, according to data provided by the Health Surveillance Agency (VISA-GO). The inclusion criteria for this study were: belonging to retail chains, medium and large supermarkets according to the IBGE classification (IBGE, 2003) (Chart 1) and having their own bakery. The exclusion criterion was frozen French bread.

Table 1. Classification of the size of Brazilian companies.

Size	**Sector** **Trade and services**
Micro	Up to 9 employees
Small	From 10 to 49 employees
Average	50 to 99 employees
Large	More than 100 employees

Source: IBGE (2003).

The following equation was used to calculate the sample size (ROSNER, 2011):

$$N = \frac{(1{,}96 \times s)^2}{e^2}$$

Where: N= Sample size;

1.96 = 95% confidence interval;

s= Standard deviation;

e= Margin of error

In order to establish the standard deviation, a pilot study was carried out by analyzing the sodium content of French bread collected from 5 bakeries in a randomly selected neighborhood in Goiânia-Goiàs, with a maximum distance of 2 km between them. Collection and analysis followed the same protocol described for this study. To determine the margin of error, we took into account the proposed 10% reduction in sodium compared to the value previously observed (324 mg of sodium/50 g of bread) (NEPA, 2011), adopting 32 mg as the margin of error.

The pilot study found the following values for sodium content (mg/ 100 g of French bread): 664 mg; 591 mg; 781 mg; 752 mg and 652 mg. The standard deviation of these values was 77.50. Using the equation (95% confidence interval, 32 mg margin of error and 77.5 mg standard deviation) the sample size was 22.53.

Thus, out of a total of 50 supermarkets that met the selection criteria for medium and large supermarkets, a representative sample of 23 locations was randomly drawn. It is worth noting that the sample included at least one establishment from each region of Goiânia-Goias.

4.3 DATA COLLECTION

Data was collected in three stages. In the first stage, four units of French bread, approximately 200g, were purchased from each of the selected supermarkets. In the second stage, bread samples were collected with the support of VISA-GO and had a maximum interval of 40 days between the first collection. At this stage, a semi-structured questionnaire (Appendix A) was administered to the baker or technical manager present in order to get to know the reality of the establishments regarding the production of French bread.

In the third stage, only samples were taken of brands of pre-mixed French bread (with variations in their formulation of wheat flour, salt and improver) used by some establishments.

It is worth noting that a maximum of five establishments were visited on each collection day and the bread collected was transported to the analysis laboratory and the analysis began on the same day.

The bread collected in both stages was weighed on a semi-analytical precision scale and the values observed were compared with the standard average weight of a portion of French bread, which corresponds to 50 g, established by RDC no. 359, of December 23, 2003 (BRASIL, 2003).

4.4 VARIABLES STUDIED

4.4.1 Questionnaire variables

Supermarket size: categorized as medium or large;

How French bread is made: categorized into own production and the use of French bread pre-mix;

Average daily production of French bread in (kg): categorized from 0 to 70 kg/day, 70 to 140 kg/day, 140 to 210 kg/day, 210 to 280 kg/day and 280 to 350 kg/day;

It has a technical file: categorized as yes or no;

The technical data sheet is used in the manufacturing process: categorized into is used by all bakers, is used by some bakers, is not used and does not apply to cases where there is no technical data sheet;

Use of the scale: categorized as yes or no;

Scale accuracy: categorized as 1 in 1g, 2 in 2g, 5 in 5g and not applicable for cases where no scale is used;

Regarding receiving training for employees: categorized as yes or no;

Length of use of current prescription: continuous and categorized into less than 1 year, 1 to 2 years, 2 to 3 years, 3 to 4 years and 5 years or more;

If there has been a change in the quantity of any ingredient in the recipe: categorized as yes, no or I can't answer;

If there has been a change of salt in the recipe: categorized as yes or no.

4.4.2 Moisture content analysis

Moisture was determined using method No. 935.36, AOAC - *The Association of Official Analytical Chemists* (2011) by dissection (at 105°C) in a drying and sterilizing oven (FANEM oven, model 315 SE, Sao Paulo, Brazil) until constant weight (variation < 0.0005 g between the last and second last weighing).

4.4.3 Sodium content analysis

All the material used during the chemical analysis of the samples was decontaminated with Stran solution for two hours and washed with milli-Q water (considered ultra-pure).

The sodium content was determined using the ash dilution method (IAL, 2008). Method no. 930.22 AOAC (2011) was used to determine the fixed mineral residue or ash. 3 g of the homogenized bread sample was weighed into a previously weighed crucible and charred over a direct flame using a Bunsen burner until it stopped smoking. After this stage, 3 drops of 65% nitric acid were added to the crucible and taken to the muffle furnace (Forno Mufla EDG 7000, Sao Carlos-SP, Brazil) for seven hours at 550°C, until the samples were completely calcined (ashes without dark spots) and constant weight, by drying in an oven at 105°C.

The ash produced and determined was transferred to a 50 mL volumetric flask, and the volume was topped up with a 1:1 (v/v) nitric acid solution (IAL, 2008). Dilution was then carried out (0.5 mL: 9.5 mL milli-Q water) to read the sodium in the flame photometer (Analyser flame photometer, model 910M, Sâo Paulo, Brazil).

The final value was determined by the average of the values converted into g Na^+ per 100g of French bread, wet basis.

The analytical parameters used to validate the determination method were linearity and the calibration curve (Figure 3) at concentrations of 20 mg/L, 40 mg/L, 60 mg/L, 80 mg/L and 100 mg/L using a stock solution (SpecSol, Brazil, 2015) of sodium at a concentration of 1000 mg/L.

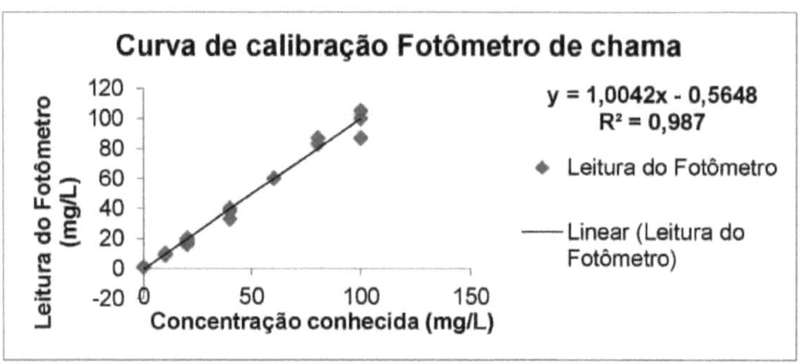

Figure 1. Calibration curve of the flame photometer studied.

The analyses were carried out in triplicate at the Food Analysis Laboratory (LANAL) of the Faculty of Nutrition of the Federal University of Goiàs (FANUT/UFG) and at the Food Quality Control Laboratory (LCQA) of the Faculty of Pharmacy of the Federal University of Goiàs (FF/UFG).

Sodium values observed above 586 mg/ 100g of French bread are not in accordance with the Term of Commitment signed between industries and the Ministry of Health (MINISTÉRIO DA SAÙDE, 2011b).

4.5 STATISTICAL ANALYSIS

The results are expressed as mean and standard deviation. The average moisture and sodium values were subjected to the normality test (Shapiro-Wilk) and *Student*'s t-test. A significance level of $p<0.05$ was adopted. Pearson's correlation was also carried out between the sodium content of the two samples and bivariate analysis was carried out between items in the bread production method and the sodium content of the samples. The statistical analyses were carried out using R software version 3.2.0 (R CORE TEAM, 2014).

4.6 ETHICAL ASPECTS

Sample collection was supported by the Municipal Health Department and VISA-GO and approved by the Research Ethics Committee of the Federal University of Goiás (Opinion number: 1.470.376; CAAE number: 51346615.4.0000.5083). The participants were informed about the research in a complete and layman's way and invited to take part after signing the Informed Consent Form (ICF) (Appendix B) to answer the questionnaire on the production of French bread, in accordance with resolution no. 466/2012 (BRASIL, 2012).

REFERENCES

ANDERSEN, L.; RASMUSSEN, L. B.; LARSEN, E. H.; JAKOBSEN, J. Intake of household salt in a Danish population. **European Journal of Clinical Nutrition**, London, v. 63, n. 5, p. 598-604, 2009.

ANVISA - National Health Surveillance Agency. Ministry of Health (Brazil). **Technical report nº 43/2010**: nutritional profile of processed foods. Brasilia, DF: ANVISA, 2010. 52 p. Available at:

<http://portal.anvisa.gov.br/wps/wcm/connect/c476ee0047457a6e86efd63fbc 4c6735/INFORME+T%C3%89CNICO+n++43+-+2010-

+PERFIL+NUTRICIONAL+_2_.pdf ?MOD=AJPERES>. Accessed on: March 23, 2015.

ANVISA - National Health Surveillance Agency. Ministry of Health (Brazil). **Guide to good nutritional practices for French bread**. Brasilia, DF: ANVISA, 2012a. Available at:

<http://portal.anvisa.gov.br/wps/wcm/connect/e3e08d8049ac9235 9467b66dcbd9c63c/Guia+de+Boas+Pr%C3%A1ticas+Nutricional+for+p% C3%A3o+franc%C3%AAs.pdf?MOD=AJPERES>. Accessed on: 25 Feb. 2015.

ANVISA - National Health Surveillance Agency. Ministry of Health (Brazil). **Technical report no *50/2012*:** sodium content of processed foods. Brasilia, DF: ANVISA, 2012b. 27 p. Available at:

<http://www.nutritotal. com.br/diretrizes/files/27 1-INFORME_TECNICO Anvisa_Processados.pdf>. Accessed on: March 23, 2015.

ANVISA - National Health Surveillance Agency. Ministry of Health (Brazil). **Technical report 542013**: sodium content of foods

processed. Brasilia, DF: ANVISA, 2013. 21 p. Available at:<http://portal.anvisa.gov.br/ wps/wcm/connect/8ab9538040695edd83fed3dc5a12ff52/INFORME+T%C3% 89CNICO+JULHO+2013.pdf?MOD=AJPERES>. Accessed on: March 23, 2015.

ANVISA - National Health Surveillance Agency. Ministry of Health (Brazil) **Technical Report no 61/2014**: sodium content in processed foods. Brasilia, DF: ANVISA, 2014. Available

em:<http://s.anvisa.gov.br/wps/wcm/connect/1e d11a004512fdc681bdf9e784b81089/INFORME+T%C3%89CNICO+N.+61+A GOSTO+2014.pdf?MOD=AJPERES>. Accessed on: March 23, 2015.

ANVISA - National Health Surveillance Agency. Ministry of Health (Brazil) **Technical Report no 69/2015**: sodium content in processed foods. Brasilia, DF: ANVISA, 2015. Available at:< http://portal.anvisa.gov.br/documents/33916/3887

29/Informe+T%C3%A9cnico+n%C2%BA+69+de+2015/85d1d8f0-5761-4195-

9aee-e992abd29b3e>. Accessed on: March 23, 2017.

AOAC- ASSOCIATION OF OFFICIAL ANALYTICAL CHEMISTS. **Official methods of analysis of the Association of Official Analytical Chemists**. Arlington: A.O.A.C., 2011, 18. ed., 4. ed. rev. 326p.

BARR, S. I. Reducing dietary sodium intake: the Canadian context. **Applied Physiology, Nutrition, and Metabolism**, Ottawa, v. 35, n. 1, p. 1-8, 2010.

BANNWART, G. C. M. C.; SILVA, M. E. M. P; VIDAL, G. Sodium reduction in foods: current panorama and technological, sensory and public health impacts. **Revista da Sociedade Brasileira de Alimentaçâo e** Nutriçâo, Sâo Paulo, v. 39, n. 3, p. 348-365, 2014.

BERTRAM, M. Y.; STEYN, K.; WENTZEL-VILJOEN, E.; TOLLMAN, S.; HOFMAN, K. J. Reducing the sodium content of high-salt foods: effect on cardiovascular disease in South Africa. **South African Medical Journal**, Cape Town, v. 102, n. 9, p. 743-745, 2012.

BOLHUIS, D. P.; TEMME, E. H. M.; KOEMAN, F. T.; NOORT, M. W. J.; KREMER, S.; JANSSEN, A. M. A salt reduction of 50% in bread does not decrease bread consumption or increase sodium intake by the choice of sandwich fillings. **The Journal of Nutrition**, Philadelphia, v. 141, n. 12, p. 2249-2255, 2011.

BRAZIL. **Resolution RDC No. 359, of December 23, 2003**. Technical regulation on portions of packaged foods for nutritional labeling purposes. Diàrio Oficial da Uniâo, Brasilia, DF, 26 dec. 2003. Available at: < http://www.abic.com.br/publique/media/CONS_leg_resolucao359-03.pdf>.

Accessed on: Aug. 10, 2016

BRAZIL. **Resolution No. 466, of December 12, 2012**. Official Journal of the Union, Brasilia, DF, June 13, 2013. Available

at:<http://conselho.saude.gov.br/resolucoes /2012/Reso466.pdf> .

Accessed

on: Aug. 23, 2016.

BRESLIN, P. A. S.; SPECTOR, A. C. Mammalian taste perception. **Current Biology**, London, v. 18, n. 4, p. R148-155, 2008.

BRINSDEN, H. C.; HE, F. J.; JENNER, K. H.; MACGREGOR, G. A. Surveys of the salt content in UK bread: progress made and further reductions possible. **BMJ Open**, London, v. 3, n. 6, p. 1-7, 2013.

BROWN, I.; TZOULAKI, I.; CANDEIAS, V.; ELLIOT, P. Salt intake worldwide: implications for public health. **International Journal of Epidemiology**, London, v. 38, n. 3, p. 791-813, 2009.

CAMPBELL, N. R. C.; JOHNSON, J. A.; CAMPBELL, T. S. Sodium consumption: an individual's choice? **International Journal of Hypertension**, London, v. 2012, p. 1-6, 2011.

CHANDRASHEKAR, J.; KUHN C.; OKA Y.; YARMOLINSKY D. A.; HUMMLER E.;. RYBA N. J. P; ZUKE C. S. The cells and peripheral representation of sodium taste in mice. **Nature**, London, v. 464, n. 7286, p. 297-301, 2010.

COBCROFT, M.; TIKELLIS, K.; BUSCH, J. L. H. C. Salt reduction: a technical overview. **Food Australia**, North Sydney, v.60, n. 3, p. 83-86, 2008.

CORDAIN, L.; EATON, S. B.; SEBASTIAN, A.; MANN, N.; LINDEBERG, S.; WATKINS, B. A.; H O'KEEFE, J.; BRAND-MILLER, J. Origins and evolution of the Western diet: health implications for the 21st[st] century. **The American Journal of Clinical Nutrition**, Bethesda, v. 81, n. 2, p. 341-354, 2005.

COOK, N. R.; CUTLER, J. A.; OBARZANEK, E.;BURING, J. E.; REXRODE, K. M.; KUMANYIKA, S. K.; APPEL, L. J.; WHELTON, P. K. Long term effects of dietary sodium reduction on cardiovascular disease outcomes: observational follow-up of the trials of hypertension prevention (TOHP). **BMJ**, London, v. 885, n. 4, p 01-08, 2007.

COTTON, P. A.; SUBAR, A. F.; FRIDAY, J. E.; COOK, A. Dietary sources of nutrients among us adults, 1994 to 1996. **Journal of the American Dietetic Association**, Chicago, v. 104, n.6, p. 921-930, 2004.

DRAKE, S. L.; DRAKE, M. A. Comparison of salty taste and time intensity of sea and land salts from around the world. **Journal of Sensory Studies**,

Malden, v. 25, n.1 p.25-34, 2011.

DOTSH, M.; BUSCH, J.; BATENBURG, M.; LIEM, G.; TAREILUS, E.; MUELLER, R.; MEIJER, G. Strategies to reduce sodium consumption: a food industry perspective. **Critical Reviews in Food Science and Nutrition**, Boca Raton, v. 49, p.841-851, 2009.

ELLIOTT, P., STAMLER, J.; NICHOLS, R.; DYER, A. R.; STAMLER, R.; KESTELOOT, H.; MARMOT, M. Intersalt revisited: further analysis of 24-hour sodium excretion and blood pressure within and across populations. **BMJ**, London, v. 312, p. 1249-1253, 1996.

FERRANTE, D.; APRO, N.; FERREIRA, V.; VIRGOLINI, M.; AGUILAR, V.; SOSA, M.; PEREL, P.; CASAS, J. Feasibility of salt reduction in processed foods in Argentina. **Revista Panamericana de Salud Pùblica**, Washington, v. 29, n. 2, p. 69-75, 2011.

FRASSETTO, L.; MORRIS JR, R. C.; SELLMEYER, D. E.; TODD, K.; SEBASTIAN, A. Diet, evolution and aging: the pathophysiologic effects of the post-agricultural inversion of the potassium-to-sodium and base-to-chloride ratios in the human diet. **European Journal of Nutrition**, Darmstadt, v. 40, n. 5, p. 200-213, 2001.

FSA - FOOD STANDARDS AGENCY. **Salt reduction targets for 2017**. United Kingdom, 2014. Available at: <http://www.food.gov.uk/northern-ireland/nutritionni/salt-ni/salt_targets>. Accessed on: August 5, 2016.

GELEIJNSE, J. M.; KOK, F. J.; GROBBEE, D. E. Blood pressure response to changes in sodium and potassium intake: a metaregression analysis of randomized trials. **Journal of Human Hypertension**, Houndmils, v.17, n. 7, p.471-80, 2003.

GIRGIS, S.; NEAL, B.; PRESCOTT, J.; DUMBRELL, S.; TURNER, C.; WOODWARD, M. A one-quarter reduction in the salt content of bread can be made without detection. **European Journal of Clinical Nutrition**, London, v.

57, n. 4, p. 616-620, 2003.

HE, F. J.; MACGREGOR, G. A. Effect of modest salt reduction on blood pressure: a meta-analysis of randomized trials. Implications for public health. **Journal of Human Hypertension**, Houndmils, v.16, n.11, p.761-70, 2002.

HE, F. J.; MACGREGOR, G. A. A comprehensive review on salt and health and current experience of worldwide salt reduction programs. **Journal of Human Hypertension**, Houndmills, v. 23, n. 6, p. 363-84, 2009.

HUTTON, T. Sodium Technological functions of salt in the manufacturing of food and drink products. **British Food Journal**, Bradford, v. 104, n. 2, p. 126152, 2002.

HOUGH G.; WAKELING, IAN, MUCCI, A., CHAMBERS IV, E., GALLARDO, I. ME'NDEZ, ALVES, L.R. Number of consumers necessary for sensory acceptability tests. **Food Quality and Preference**, Barking, v.17, p. 522-526, 2006.

IAL - ADOLF LUTZ INSTITUTE. ZENEBON. **Physico-chemical methods for food analysis**. Sao Paulo: Instituto Adolfo Lutz, 2008. 1. ed. online, 1020p. Available: <http://www.crq4.org.br/sms/files/file/analisedealimentosial_2008.pdf>. Accessed on: 25 Feb. 2015.

IBGE - BRAZILIAN INSTITUTE OF GEOGRAPHY AND STATISTICS. **Family budget survey 2008-2009**: household food purchases per capita: Brazil and Major Regions. Rio de Janeiro: IBGE, 2010. 276 p. Available at : <http://www.ibge.gov.br/home/estatistica/populacao/condicaodevida/pof/2008_2009_aquisicao/pof20082009_aquisicao.pdf>. Accessed on: 25 Feb. 2015.

IBGE - BRAZILIAN INSTITUTE OF GEOGRAPHY AND STATISTICS. **Micro and small commercial and service companies in Brazil**: 2001. IBGE, Coordination of Services and Trade: Rio de Janeiro, 2003. 100p.

KoTCHEN, T. A.; CoWLEY, A. W.; FRoHLIC, E. D. salt in health and disease: a delicate balance. **New England Journal of Medicine**, Boston, v. 368, n. 13, p. 1229-1237, 2013.

LA CRoIX, K. W.; FIALA, s. C.; CoLoNNA, A. E.; DURHAM, C. A.; MoRRIssEY, M. T.; DRUM, D. K.; KoHN, M. A. Consumer detection and acceptability of reduced-sodium bread. **Public Health Nutrition**, Wallingford, v. 18, n. 8, p. 1412-1418, 2015.

LIEM, D. G.; MIREMADI, F.; KEAST, R. s. J. Reducing sodium in foods: the effect on flavor. **Nutrients**, Basel, v. 3, n. 6, p. 694-711, 2011.

LYNCH, E. J.; BELLo, F. D.; sHEEHAN, E. M.; CAsHMAN, K. D.; ARENDT, E. K. Fundamental studies on the reduction of salt on dough and bread characteristics. **Food Research International**, Toronto, v. 42, p. 885-891, 2009.

MAN, C. M. D. Technological functions of salt in food products. In: Kilcast D, Angus F, editors. **Reducing salt in foods**: practical strategies. Cambridge: Woodhead, 2007. p. 157-73.

MCLEAN, R. M. Measuring population sodium intake: a review of methods. **Nutrients**, Basel, v. 6, n. 11, p. 4651-4662, 2014.

MENEToN, P.; JEUNEMAITRE, X.; DE WARDENER, H. E.; MACGREGoR, G. A. Links between dietary salt intake, renal salt handling, blood pressure, and cardiovascular diseases. **Physiological Reviews**, Bethesda, v. 85, n. 2, p. 679-715, 2005.

MHURCHU, N. C.; CAPELIN, C.; DUNFORD, E. K.; WEBSTER, J. L.; NEAL, B. C.; JEBB, S. A. Sodium content of processed foods in the United Kingdom: analysis of 44,000 foods purchased by 21,000 households. **The American Journal of Clinical Nutrition**, Bethesda, v. 93, n. 3, p. 594-600, 2011.

MICHELL, A. R. **The clinical biology of sodium**: the physiology and pathophysiology of sodium in mammals. Oxford: Elsevier Science, 1995. 388

p.

MINISTRY OF HEALTH. Secretariat of Health Care, Department of Primary Health Care. **Food guide for the Brazilian population**. Brasilia: Ministry of Health; 2014. Available at: http://foodpolitics.com/wp- content/uploads/Brazils-Dietary-Guidelines_2014.pdf . Accessed on: 02 Aug 2016.

MINISTRY OF HEALTH. Secretariat of Health Care, Department of Basic Care. **National Food and Nutrition Policy**. Brasilia: Ministry of Health; 2012. (Series B. Textos Bàsicos de Saùde). Available at: <http://189.28.128.100/nutricao/docs/geral/pnan2011.pdf>. Accessed on: March 23, 2015.

MINISTRY OF HEALTH. Health Surveillance Secretariat, Health Situation Analysis Department. **Strategic action plan for tackling chronic non-communicable diseases in Brazil 2011 - 2022**. Brasilia: Ministry of Health, 2011a. 148 p.

MINISTRY OF HEALTH. Commitment agreement between the Ministry of Health and the Brazilian Food Industry Association (ABIA), the Brazilian Pasta Industry Association (ABIMA), the Brazilian Wheat Industry Association (ABITRIGO) and the Brazilian Bakery and Confectionery Industry Association (ABIP) with the aim of establishing national targets for reducing the sodium content in processed foods in Brazil. Brasilia - DF. 2011. In: **Diàrio Oficial da Uniâo** -DOU, section 3, page 124. 26 Dec 2011b. Available at: <http://189.28.128.100/dab/docs/portaldab/documentos/termo_5_dez_2011.pdf.> Accessed on: 12 Jan 2015.

MORRIS, M. J.; NA, E. S.; JOHNSON, A. K. Salt craving: the psychobiology of pathogenic sodium intake. **Physiology & Behavior**, Elmsford, v. 94, n. 5, p. 709-721, 2008.

NATIONAL CENTER FOR SOCIAL RESEARCH. **An assessment of dietary**

sodium levels among adults (aged 19-64) in the general population in Wales, based on analysis of dietary sodium in 24-hour urine samples. 2007. Available at at:<http://webarchive.nationalarchives.gov.uk/20101211052406/http:/www.food.gov.uk/multimedia/pdfs/walessodiumreport.pdf.>. Accessed on: 19 Jun 2015

NEPA - Nùcleo de Estudos Aplicados em Nutriçâo. UNICAMP. TACO - **Brazilian food composition table**. 4. ed. 161p. Campinas, UNICAMP, 2011. Available at: <http://www.unicamp.br/ nepa/taco/contar/taco_4_edicao_ampliada_e_revisada>. Accessed on: September 30, 2015.

NILSON, E. A. F.; JAIME, P. C.; RESENDE, D. O. Initiatives developed in Brazil to reduce sodium content in processed foods. **Revista Panamericana de Salud Pùblica**, Washington, v. 34 n. 4, p.287-292, 2012.

NWANGUMA, B. C.; OKORIE, C. H. Salt (sodium chloride) content of retail samples of Nigerian white bread: implications for the daily salt intake of normotensive and hypertensive adults. **Journal of Human Nutrition and Dietetics**, London, v. 26, n. 5, p. 488-493, 2013.

OBLIGADO, S. H.; GOLDFARB, D. S. The association of nephrolithiasis with hypertension and obesity: a review. **American Journal of Hypertension**, New York, v. 21, n. 3, p. 257-264, 2008.

PAGE, L. B.; DAMON, A.; MOELLERING, R. C. Antecedents of cardiovascular disease in six Solomon islands societies. **Circulation**, Dallas, v. 49, n. 6, p. 1132-1146, 1974.

PFEIFFER, C. M.; HUGHES, J. P.; COGSWELL, M. E.; BURT, V. L.;LACHER, D. A.; LAVOIE, D. J.; RABINOWITZ, D. J.; JOHNSON, C. L.; PIRKLE, J. L. Urine sodium excretion increased slightly among U.S. adults between 1988 and 2010. **The Journal of Nutrition**, Philadelphia, v. 144, n. 5, p. 698-705,

2014.

POTTER, P. A.; PERRY; [translated by Luciana Teixeira Gomes; Lucia Helena Duarte; Maria Inês Correa Nascimento]. **Fundamentals of nursing**. 6. ed. Rio de Janeiro: Elsevier, 2005. 1.729 p.

R CORE TEAM. **R: a Language and environment for statistical computing**. The R Foundation for Statistical Computing, Vienna, Austria, 2014.

RITZ, E. The history of salt. Aspects of interest to the nephrologist. **Nephrology Dialysis Transplantation**, Oxford, v. 11, n. 6, p. 969-975, 1996.

ROSNER, B. **Fundamentals of biostatistics**. 7. ed. Brooks/Cole: Cengage Learning, 2011. 888 p.

SARNO, F.; CLARO, R. M.; LEVY, R. B.; BANDONI, D. H.; MONTEIRO, C. A. Estimated sodium consumption by the Brazilian population, 2008-2009. **Revista de Saùde Pùblica**, Sâo Paulo, v. 47, n. 3, p. 571-578, 2013.

SCHMIDLIN, O.; FORMAN, A.; SEBASTIAN, A.; MORRIS, R. C. What initiates the pressor effect of salt in sensitive humans? Observations in normosensitive blacks. **Hypertension**, Dallas, v. 49, n. 5, p. 1032-1039, 2007.

STAMLER, J.; ELLIOT, P.; APPEL, L.; CHAN, Q.; BUZZARD, M.; DENNIS, B.; et al. Higher blood pressure in middle-aged American adults with less education-role of multiple dietary factors: the INTERMAP Study. **Journal of Human Hypertension**, Houndmills, v. 17, n. 9, p. 655-664, 2003a.

STAMLER, J.; ELLIOT, P.; DENNIS, B.; DYER, A. R.; KESTELOOT, H.; LIU, K.; et al. INTERMAP: background, aims, design, methods, and descriptive statistics (nondietary). **Journal of Human Hypertension**, Houndmills, v. 17, n. 9, p. 591-608, 2003b.

STAMLER, J. The INTERSALT Study: background, methods, findings, and implications. **The American Journal of Clinical Nutrition**, Bethesda, v. 65, n. 2, p. 626S-642, 1997.

STRAZZULLO, P.; LECLERCQ, C. Sodium. **Advances in Nutrition**, Bethesda, v. 5, n. 2, p. 188-190, 2014.

TAVARES, A; JUNIOR KOHLMANN, O. Treatment of hypertension: the value of reducing salt intake. **Hipertensâo**, Sâo Paulo, v. 7, n. 2, p. 7173, 2004.

TEKOL, Y. Salt addiction: a different kind of drug addiction. **Medical Hypothesis**, Edinburgh, v. 67, n. 5, p. 1233-1234, 2006.

TSUGANE, S.; SASAZUKI, S.; KOBAYASHI, M.; SASAKI, S. Salt and salted food intake and subsequent risk of gastric cancer among middle-aged Japanese men and women. **British Journal of Cancer**, London, v. 90, n. 1, p. 128-134, 2004.

USDA - US Department of Agriculture, US Department of health and human services. **Dietary guidelines for Americans**, 2010. 7. ed. Washington, DC: US Government Printing Office, 2010.

VALENZUELA L., K.; QUITRAL R., V; ZAVALA M. F; VILLANUEVA, A., B; ATALAH S., E. Evaluación de la aceptabilidad del pan reducido en sodio en consumidores de la Región Metropolitana de Chile. **Revista Chilena de Nutrición**, Santiago, v. 41, n. 1, p. 67-71, 2014.

VIEIRA E.; OLIVEIRA B.M.P.M.; SOARES M.E.; PINHO O. Study of sodium content in bread consumed in Porto. **Revista de Alimentaçâo Humana**, Porto, v.13, n.3, p. 97-103, 2007.

VIGITEL BRAZIL 2014. **Surveillance of risk and protective factors for chronic diseases by telephone survey**, 2014. Available at:< http://portalsaude.saude.gov.br/images/ pdf/2015/abril/15/PPT-Vigitel-2014-.pdf>. Accessed on: 20 Nov. 2016.

WEBSTER, J. L.; DUNFORD, E. K.; HAWKES, C.; NEAL, B. C. Salt reduction initiatives around the world. **Journal of Hypertension**, London, v. 29, n. 6, p. 1043-1050, 2011.

WHO - WORLD HEALTH ORGANIZATION. **Global strategy on diet, physical activity and health**. Geneva: World Health Organization, 2004. Available at: < http://www.who.int/dietphysicalactivity/strategy/eb11344/strategy_english_web.pdf> Accessed on: 12 Jan. 2015.

WHO - WORLD HEALTH ORGANIZATION. **Guideline**: sodium intake for adults and children. Geneva: WHO Library Cataloguing-in-Publication Data; 2012, reprinted 2014. Available at: < http://apps.who.int/iris/bitstream/10665/7 7985/1/9789241504836_eng.pdf> Accessed: June 18, 2015.

WHO - WORLD HEALTH ORGANIZATION. **Reducing salt intake in populations**. Report of a WHO Forum and Technical Meeting, 5-7 October 2006, Paris, France. Geneva: WHO Document Production Services, 2007. Available at: < http://www.who.int/dietphysicalactivity/reducingsaltintake_EN.pdf> Accessed on: 12 Jan. 2015.

CHAPTER 2 - SCIENTIFIC ARTICLE 1

Title: French bread production in supermarket bakeries: voluntary agreement to reduce sodium content

Short title: Sodium in French bread from supermarket bakeries

Authors: Thais Braga de Paula[1]

[1] Postgraduate Program in Nutrition and Health, Faculty of Nutrition, Universidade Federal de Goiàs, Goiânia, Goiàs, Brazil.

Sources of funding: Master's degree scholarship/CAPES awarded to Paula TB.

The author declares no conflict of interest.

SUMMARY

The aim of the study was to analyze the sodium content and production method of French bread made in supermarket bakeries in a Brazilian capital, with a view to assessing compliance with the voluntary sodium reduction agreement. This is an analytical observational cross-sectional study carried out on a representative sample of 23 medium and large supermarkets selected by random drawing. Two samples of French bread were taken and the sodium content was analyzed in the laboratory using dry digestion, dilution in acid and flame photometer readings. Qualitative aspects of how the bread was produced were analyzed using a semi-structured questionnaire. The sodium content ranged from 286 to 702 mg/100 g of bread. Only two supermarkets had bread samples above 586 mg/100g, the maximum reference value stipulated by the voluntary agreement. Of the samples analyzed, 82.6% weighed more than 50g per unit. According to the bivariate analysis, supermarkets that use their own recipes produce bread with a significantly lower sodium content than those that use ready-made premixes. Those that reduced the salt in the recipe (n=5) had bread with a lower sodium content. The voluntary agreement was complied with in 91.3% of the sites studied, with no statistical difference between the samples. However, as 78% of the stores reported that they had not changed their recipes, it can be inferred that they were already producing bread with levels in line with the agreement, which shows that the reduction targets were inadequate for bread produced in supermarkets in the capital. The bread units weighed more than recommended, leading to higher than expected sodium consumption.

Key words: sodium chloride in the diet, food preparation, salt, technology.

Introduction

According to a report by the World Health Organization (WHO), chronic non-communicable diseases (NCDs) are the leading cause of death in the world. In Brazil, they are responsible for 72% of deaths[1] , but their impact can be reversed by comprehensive health promotion measures .[2]

Among the measures is the reduction of salt in the diet, as its excess consumption is associated with an increased risk of various chronic diseases, such as hypertension and cardiovascular disease, diabetes, osteoporosis and reduced bone density, alongside other factors such as obesity, smoking and a sedentary lifestyle .[3,4]

With the aim of promoting the development and implementation of effective and sustainable public policies for the prevention and control of NCDs and risk factors, the Ministry of Health has launched the "Strategic Action Plan for Tackling NCDs in Brazil from 2011 to 2022". Among the national targets proposed for healthier eating and the prevention of CNCDs is the reduction of the average salt intake by the population through agreements with the food industry to reduce the salt content in their products and improve access to less salty processed foods .[5]

In this context, the Ministry of Health, the Brazilian Association of Food Industries (ABIA), the Brazilian Association of Pasta Industries (ABIMA), the Brazilian Wheat Industry Association (ABITRIGO) and the Brazilian Bakery and

Confectionery Industry Association (ABIP) signed a Commitment Agreement in 2011 to reduce the salt content in various products, including French bread, by the end of 2014 .[6]

French bread is present in Brazilian eating habits with an average consumption of one unit per day[7] , which is around 324 mg/ 50 g of bread (648 mg/100 g of bread), according to 2011 data from the Brazilian Food Composition Table[8] . This consumption contributes 16% of the recommended daily sodium requirement (2000 mg) - .[89]

The Term of Commitment proposed a gradual reduction in sodium content to a maximum of 586 mg of sodium/100 g of French bread by 2014, i.e. a reduction of around 10%[6] . With this reduction, the consumption of one unit of French bread (50 g) would correspond to 14.6% of the daily sodium requirement, instead of 16%.

The latest monitoring of sodium content published to date by the National Health Surveillance Agency (ANVISA) included foods from the second agreement signed, including French bread[10] . The results of these analyses included 39 samples of bread from 19 different states, including Goiás. The average sodium content found in French bread was 736 mg/100g, with results ranging from 411 mg to 880 mg. The analyses for this monitoring were carried out in 2014 and the sodium values forecast for the end of 2012 were used as targets, which were 616 mg/100g of bread[6] . It is important to note that the states were not identified when presenting the sodium levels found.

In view of this, the aim of this study was to analyze the sodium content and production method of French bread produced in supermarket bakeries in the municipality of Goiânia-Goiàs and thus assess, through the representative sample selected, compliance with the latest Term of Commitment signed by various food/bakery industry associations and the Ministry of Health, to reduce the salt content in processed foods.

Although scientific evidence from the results observed in developed countries indicates that salt reduction policies focused on processed foods may be feasible at the population level, data on the effectiveness and impact of these interventions remain limited and outdated in developing countries, such as Brazil .[11]

Methods

This is an analytical observational cross-sectional study carried out in the municipality of Goiânia, state of Goiás, located in the Center-West region of Brazil (latitude: 16° 40' 43", longitude: 49° 15' 14"), whose Human Development Index is 0.799, which is equivalent to high development.

In Goiânia, there were 344 regularized supermarkets in 2015, according to data provided by the Health Surveillance Agency (VISA-GO). The inclusion criteria for this study were: belonging to retail chains, being medium or large-sized according to the classification of the Brazilian Institute of Geography and Statistics (IBGE)[12] and having their own bakery. The exclusion criterion was the sale of French bread made from frozen bread from other suppliers.

To calculate the sample size, we used a pilot study to find out the sodium content of bread, which was carried out in five bakeries in a randomly selected neighborhood in Goiânia-Goiàs, with a maximum distance of two km between them. Collection and analysis followed the same protocol described for this study. A range of 591 to 781 mg of sodium per 100 g of bread was observed, corresponding to an average value of 688 mg ± 77.5. The value of this standard deviation was used in the sample calculation[13] . To determine the margin of error, we took into account the proposed 10% reduction in sodium compared to the value previously observed (324 mg of sodium/ 50 g of bread)[8] , thus adopting 32 mg as the margin of error. A 95% confidence interval was used.

Thus, according to the parameters: 32 mg margin of error, 77.5 mg standard deviation and 95% confidence, a sample size of 22.53 establishments was found from the population of supermarket bakeries that met the selection criteria. From a total of 50 supermarkets that met the selection criteria, a representative sample of 23 sites was randomly drawn.

Data collection

Data was collected in three stages between October 2015 and January 2016, with a maximum interval of 40 days. In the first stage, four units of French bread, approximately 200g, were purchased from each of the selected supermarkets. In the second stage, samples were taken with the support of VISA-GO. In addition, a semi-structured questionnaire was administered to the baker or technical manager present in order to find out about the reality of the establishments with regard to aspects of French bread production.

In the third stage, samples were taken of the French bread premix (with variations in its formulation of wheat flour, salt and improver) used by some establishments.

A maximum of five establishments were visited on each collection day and the bread collected was immediately taken to the laboratory and analyzed.

Weight of feet

All the bread collected was weighed on a semi-analytical scale with a precision of 0.001 g and the values observed were compared with the standard average weight of a portion of French bread, which corresponds to 50 g, as established by RDC 359/2003 .[14]

Laboratory analysis of moisture and sodium content

Moisture was determined using the dissection method (at 105°C) in a drying and sterilizing oven (FANEM oven, model 315 SE, Sâo Paulo, Brazil) until constant weight (variation < 0.0005 g between the last and second last weighing), in 935.36, AOAC - *The Association of Official Analytical Chemists* (2011) .[15]

To determine the sodium content, aliquots of the bread and premix samples were subjected to the dry digestion method of the organic matter (carbonization in a flame and calcination of the sample in a muffle furnace at 550°C), according to the ash determination procedure by method no. 930.22[15] and were transferred to a 50 mL volumetric flask, completing the volume with a 1:1 (v/v) nitric acid solution[16] . Afterwards, a new dilution was made, sample: milli-Q water, (1.0:19.0) to read the sodium in the flame photometer (Analyser Flame Photometer, model 910M, Sao Paulo, Brazil). The final value was determined by the average of the values converted into g Na+ per 100g of French bread, wet base.

The analytical parameters used to validate the determination method were: linearity and the calibration curve at concentrations of 20 mg/L, 40mg/L, 60 mg/L, 80 mg/L and 100 mg/L based on a stock solution (SpecSol, Brazil, 2015) of sodium at a concentration of 1000 mg/L. All the material used during the chemical analysis of the samples was decontaminated with a solution of Estran for two hours and rinsed with milli-Q water.

The sodium content of bread was also analyzed according to two classifications, an international one (Food Standards Agency, FSA)[17] and a state one (State Law n-19.289/ 2016)[18] and according to the maximum limit established by voluntary agreement and Term of Commitment signed between industries and the Ministry of Health .[6]

Variables studied

Data collected through direct interviews and questionnaires included: size of the supermarket (categorized as medium and large); autonomy of French bread production (categorized as own production, using own recipe and use of ready-made French bread pre-mix, with only water and yeast added); average daily production of French bread in (kg) (categorized from 0 to 70 kg/day, 70 to 140 kg/day, 140 to 210 kg/day, 210 to 280 kg/day and 280 to 350 kg/day); whether the site has a technical data sheet (categorized as yes or no); whether the technical data sheet is used in the manufacturing process (categorized as used by all bakers, used by some bakers, not used or not applicable for cases where there is no technical data sheet); whether the site uses a scale when making bread (categorized as yes or no); how accurate the scale is (categorized as 1 in 1g, 2 in 2g, 5 in 5g and not applicable for cases where no scale is used); whether there is training for employees (categorized as yes or no); how long the current recipe has been used (continuous and categorized as less than 1 year, 1 to 2 years, 2 to 3 years, 3 to 4 years and 5 years or more); whether there have been any changes to the quantity of any ingredient in the recipe since the program was implemented (categorized as yes, no and I can't answer) and whether there have been any changes to the salt in the recipe (categorized as yes or no).

Statistical analysis and ethical aspects

The results were expressed as mean and sample standard deviation. The average moisture and sodium values were subjected to the normality test (Shapiro-Wilk) and Student's t-test. A significance level of $p<0.05$ was adopted. Pearson's correlation was tested between the sodium content of the two samples and a bivariate analysis was carried out between items in the bread production method and the sodium content of the samples. The statistical analyses were carried out using R software version 3.2.0.

The sample collection work was supported by the Municipal Health Department and VISA-GO and approved by the Research Ethics Committee of the Federal University of Goiás under opinion 1.470.376. It complied with the rules for conducting research with human beings, according to CNS Resolution 466/2012[19] and the interviews were only carried out after signing the Informed Consent Form.

Results

In relation to the weight analysis of the bread, it was observed that the average weight between the units of the samples collected varied from 45.88 g to 72.13 g. 17.4% of the bread analyzed weighed between 45 and 50 g, 43.0% between 57 and 62 g, 13.0% between 63 and 68 g. Of these, 17.4% weighed between 45 and 50 g, 43.5% between 51 and 56 g, 13.0% between 57 and 62 g, 13.0%

between 63 and 68 g and 13.0% between 69 and 74 g. Thus, 82.6% of the French bread units analyzed weighed more than 50 g per unit.

As for moisture, the average values observed in the two bread collections ranged from 19.42 g/100 g to 32.38 g/100 g. The second collection obtained slightly larger samples in 14 of the supermarkets studied, but when considering the overall average of all the samples for the two collections, there was no significant difference using the t-test ($p = 0.332$) (Table 1).

The sodium content of the bread samples studied in the 23 supermarkets, considering the two collections, varied between 286 mg/100 g and 702 mg/100 g of bread (corresponding to 0.72 g salt/100 g and 1.76 g salt/100 g). The average value found was 465 mg sodium/100 g bread (corresponding to 1.16 g salt/100 g) with a standard deviation of 97.9 mg sodium/100 g (Table 1).

Table 1. Average values and standard deviation of moisture and sodium content of French bread samples, in the two collections from October 2015 to January 2016 (wet basis).

Supermarket	**Moisture (mg/100 g)**			**Sodium content (mg/ 100 g)**		
	1ª collection	**2nd collection**	**Average**	**1st collection**	**2nd collection**	**Average**
A	27,9 ± 0,2*	28,6 ± 0,2	28,3 ± 0,5	511 ± 0,0	556 ± 0,0	534 ± 31,7
B	23,0 ± 0,2	24,0 ± 0,2	23,5 ± 0,7	589 ± 0,0	669 ± 0,0	629 ± 56,4
C	27,7 ± 0,2	25,2 ± 0,1	26,4 ± 1,8	421 ± 0,0	455 ± 0,0	438 ± 23,9
D	20,4 ± 0,2	28,4 ± 0,2	24,4 ± 5,7	601 ± 0,0	544 ± 0,0	573 ± 40,4
E	26,7 ± 0,1	29,5 ± 0,1	28,1 ± 2,0	532 ± 0,0	500 ± 0,0	516 ± 22,7
F	29,6 ± 0,3	31,7 ± 0,2	30,7 ± 1,5	324 ± 6,5	387 ± 0,0	355 ± 44,9
G	29,9 ± 0,3	29,2 ± 0,3	29,6 ± 0,5	286 ± 0,0	387 ± 0,0	337 ± 71,7
H	28,6 ± 0,1	27,2 ± 0,2	27,9 ± 1,0	286 ± 0,0	511 ± 0,0	398 ± 159,4
I	25,6 ± 0,1	27,9 ± 0,2	26,7 ± 1,6	399 ± 0,0	466 ± 0,0	432 ± 47,0
J	26,7 ± 0,0	30,3 ± 0,3	28,5 ± 2,5	354 ± 0,0	455 ± 0,0	405 ± 71,7
K	27,5 ± 0,2	22,8 ± 0,3	25,2 ± 3,3	442 ± 0,0	365 ± 0,0	403 ± 54,2
L	24,3 ± 0,7	27,0 ± 0,1	25,7 ± 1,9	615 ± 25,9	555 ± 0,0	585 ± 42,4
M	30,2 ± 0,2	26,8 ± 0,3	28,5 ± 2,4	397 ± 11,2	398 ± 0,0	397 ± 0,5
N	26,2 ± 0,4	32,4 ± 0,2	29,3 ± 4,4	309 ± 0,0	399 ± 0,0	354 ± 63,6

O	25,8 ± 0,3	31,5 ± 0,4	28,6 ± 4,1	365 ± 0,0	387 ± 0,0	376 ± 16,1
P	19,4 ± 0,2	22,2 ± 0,2	20,8 ± 2,0	702 ± 0,0	634 ± 0,0	668 ± 48,1
Q	28,8 ± 0,1	29,9 ± 0,1	29,4 ± 0,8	511 ± 0,0	579 ± 0,0	545 ± 47,9
R	26,2 ± 0,2	29,4 ± 0,2	27,8 ± 2,2	350 ± 0,0	308 ± 0,0	329 ± 29,5
S	29,6 ± 0,2	23,8 ± 0,2	26,7 ± 4,1	399 ± 0,0	376 ± 0,0	388 ± 16,1
T	28,4 ± 0,1	28,7 ± 0,2	28,6 ± 0,2	447 ± 0,0	556 ± 0,0	502 ± 77,3
U	25,6 ± 0,2	22,0 ± 0,1	23,8 ± 2,6	346 ± 6,5	590 ± 0,0	468 ± 172,1
V	28,4 ± 0,3	28,0 ± 0,2	28,2 ± 0,3	500 ± 0,0	600 ± 0,0	550 ± 70,5
X	30,5 ± 0,1	30,0 ± 0,2	30,2 ± 0,4	530 ± 26,0	511 ± 0,0	521 ± 13,1
Total*	26,8 ± 2,9	27,7 ± 3,0	27,3 ± 1,5	444 ± 115,1	486 ± 98,3	465 ± 97,9
T-test for all data		p= 0,332			p= 0,187	

* Values expressed as mean and sample standard deviation.

A positive correlation of good magnitude was observed between the sodium content of the two collections (R= 068, p < 0.001). In addition, a paired t-test was carried out between the sodium content found in the 1ª collection and the 2ª collection and no statistical difference was observed between the collections (p = 0.187).

When considering the maximum reference value of 586 mg of sodium/100 g of bread, defined in the voluntary agreement[6] , only two supermarkets (B and P) were above this value in relation to the averages of the two samples.

Data from the different classifications of the sodium content of the bread analyzed are shown in Table 2.

Table 2. Distribution of supermarkets by range of average sodium content in bread, observed in the two collections (mg/100g) (n=23).

Average sodium content (mg/100g bread)	Supermarkets n	%	Classification according to State Law no. 19.289, of May 4, 2016	Classification according to FSA*, 2012
[300 - 400[	8	34,8	34.8 % below 400	
[400 - 500[	5	21,7	mg	91.3 % below

				600 mg
[500 - 600[	8	34,8	65.2 % with high sodium content	
[600 - 700[	2	8,7		8.7 % with high sodium content

*FSA - Food Standards Agency

In terms of how French bread is produced, 69.6% of the supermarkets studied are medium-sized and the majority (65.2%) make their own bread. The remainder (34.8%) use a pre-mix for French bread (Table 3), in which they usually only add water and biological yeast. The bakers mentioned using seven different brands of premix.

Table 3. Data on the production method of French bread in the supermarkets studied. (n=23).

Items evaluated	N	%
Size of the supermarket		
Medium	16	69,6
Large	7	30,4
Manufacturing		
Own production	15	65,2
Use of premix	8	34,8
Quantity of French bread produced/day		
0 to 70 kg/day	4	17,4
70 to 140 kg/day	8	34,8
140 to 210 kg/day	5	21,7
210 to 280 kg/day	3	13
280 to 350 kg/day	3	13
It has a technical sheet		
Yes	19	82,6
No	4	17,4
Using the data sheet		

All the bakers	19	82,6
Not applicable	4	17,4
Use of scales		
Yes	21	91,3
No	2	8,7
Scale accuracy		
1 in 1g	7	30,4
2 in 2g	4	17,4
5 in 5g	10	43,5
Not applicable	2	8,7
Training		
Yes	22	95,6
No	1	4,4
Recipe usage time		
Less than 1 year	1	4,4
Between 1 and 2 years	1	4,4
Between 2 and 3 years	3	13
Between 3 and 4 years	7	30,4
5 years or more	11	47,8
Changing an ingredient in the recipe		
Yes	5	21,8
No	16	69,6
Couldn't answer	2	8,7
Change the salt in the recipe		
Yes	5	21,8
No	18	78,2

In terms of the amount of French bread produced per day, 56.5% produce between 70 and 210 kg, and 26% between 210 and 350 kg, i.e. between 1,400 and 7,000 units per day.

Among the supermarkets, 82.6% said they had a technical sheet for preparing French bread and all of them reported that the sheet is used by all the bakers, i.e. on all shifts. With regard to the scales, 91.3% use them when preparing bread, with 43.5% being accurate to 5g. With regard to training in the standardized preparation of bread, 95.6% of the sites reported that employees receive it.

When asked how long they had been using the current recipe, 47.8% had been using it for 5 years or more and 30.4% had been using it for between 3 and 4 years, i.e., according to the reports, the majority of stores had not changed the recipe as a result of the Commitment Agreement, and had not reduced the amount of salt in the original recipe. Only five supermarkets (21.8%) said they had reduced the salt in the recipe, four of which were from the same chain.

Bivariate analysis was carried out between each item assessed in the questionnaire and the sodium content of the bread analyzed. A significant association was found only between the way in which the bread is made (whether it is made in-house or uses pre-mix) and whether the supermarket has changed the amount of salt in the recipe (Figure 1).

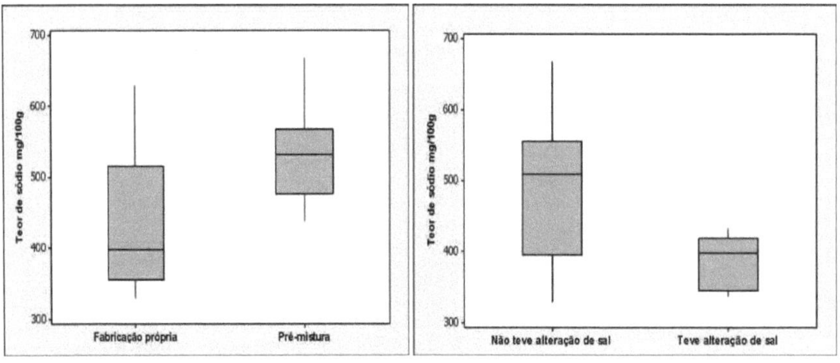

Manufacturing	Average values and standard deviation of sodium/100 g of bread	Change the salt in the recipe	Average values and standard deviation of sodium/100 g of bread
In-house production	429 ± 92,6	Yes (n=5)	385 ± 39,1

(n=15)			
Use of premix	533 ± 70,3	No (n=18)	488 ± 98,2
(n=8)	p = 0,001		p= 0,006
Grand total	**465 ± 98**	**Grand total**	**465±98**

Figure 1. Graphical representation of the comparison between sodium content, method of manufacture and change of salt in the recipe.

In addition, an analysis was carried out of the seven brands of pre-mix for French bread mentioned by the establishments. According to the labeling, 30 to 50 g of pre-mix are needed to make a 50 g loaf of French bread, depending on the brand. Two brands (5, 7) exceeded the maximum sodium content defined in the voluntary agreement for 100 g of bread (Table 4).

Table 4: Sodium content of different brands of premix in 100g of premix and

100g of bread (produced according to the portion indicated by the manufacturer on the label).

Brand	Sodium content in 10i) g of premix*	Sodium content in 100 g of ready-made French bread**
1	396 ± 11,2	396 mg/ 100 g of bread produced with 100 g of premix
2	673 ± 0,0	538 mg/ 100 g of bread produced with 80 g of premix
3	703 ± 6,5	562 mg/ 100 g of bread produced with 80 g of premix
4	860 ± 0,0	516 mg/ 100 g of bread produced with 60 g of premix
5	748 ± 13,0	**598 mg/ 100 g of bread** produced with 80 g of premix
6	330 ± 0,0	330 mg/ 100 g of bread produced with 100 g of premix
7	636 ± 0,0	**636 mg/ 100 g of bread** produced with 100 g of premix

* Values were determined in a laboratory and expressed as mean and sample standard deviation, ** as indicated for the production of 100 g of bread. In bold, brands that exceeded the target of the voluntary sodium reduction agreement.

Discussion

Currently, in Brazil, there is no legislation that determines what the weight of a unit of French bread should be, since it is currently marketed by weight.

However, the ideal average weight is 50g for a unit, which corresponds to 150 kcal for a portion, according to the recommendations for bakery products, cereals, legumes, roots and tubers, and their derivatives by Resolution RDC No. 359 of December 23, 2003[14] . Observing that most of the supermarkets studied produce bread heavier than 50g, the sodium content consumed may be higher than expected since bread is consumed per unit and not by weight.

For example, in the supermarket "Q", whose bread has an average of 545 mg sodium/100 g of bread (within the recommendation, < 586 mg/100g), and an average weight of 70 g of bread, a single unit consumed by an individual contributes 381.5 mg of sodium at one time, which corresponds to 19.1% of the daily sodium requirement (analysis of consumption of pure bread without filling).

Therefore, as educational and preventive measures for the health of the population, in relation to the consumption of salt/sodium per unit of bread, greater standardization of bread size is suggested as an important strategy. In addition, differences in the weight of bread units negatively affect the work of health professionals, such as nutritionists, who work with home measurements and calculate and prescribe the consumption of bread within the recommended portion weight, i.e. 50 g per unit .[20]

With regard to moisture, in the Brazilian regulations for the standard of identity and quality of French bread, only Resolution RDC no 90, of October 18, 2000, which has now been revoked, mentioned a maximum moisture content of 38% for French bread, considering the dough free of toppings and fillings. However, the current resolution, RDC no. 263, of September 22, 2005[21] , removed this determination on the maximum moisture content. No moisture content limits were observed in international resolutions. However, none of the samples studied had a moisture content above 38%. It is worth noting that moisture analysis was carried out in this study to determine the best way of comparing sodium content. As there was no statistical difference between the breads from different establishments and collections, it was possible to compare the sodium content on a wet basis, the form presented in most scientific articles on sodium in breads.

According to the sodium content classifications, the bread analyzed can be designated in various ways, depending on the regulatory body. The UK classification[17] considers high sodium content when there is more than 600 mg/ 100 g of food. This classification is less rigorous and according to it a small proportion of the breads studied are high in sodium.

In Goiás, Brazil, State Law No. 19.289, of May 4, 2016[18] , defined as mandatory the indication of which foods have a high sodium content on the menus of restaurants, bars and the like (≥ 400 mg of sodium/100 g of food). According to this classification, most of the bread analyzed has a high sodium content and therefore establishments should indicate the classification of the bread (high content) to their consumers, which has not been done. The state regulation is in line with other public policies[23-25] to encourage the creation of healthy eating habits by the population from childhood onwards, with the state duly involved in protecting this right to adequate food, when necessary. However, as an effective measure for consumers, it is recommended that the data also be expressed in a household measure, as is done in food labeling.

According to the criteria of the PAHO (Pan American Health Organization) Nutritional Profile Model[22] , a processed or multiprocessed food contains excess sodium when the ratio between the amount of sodium in a given quantity and the energy value is greater than or equal to 1. In this sense, if we consider that 100g of French bread has around 300 kcal[8] , when we evaluate the breads studied according to this energy value, they all have excessive sodium content.

With regard to the method of manufacture, it is valid to say that the use of pre-mixes for French bread is a trend in the market, as they reduce costs, reduce the stock of raw materials, standardize product quality and make better use of the workforce, as it is not necessary to weigh the ingredients individually 26. Some brands of pre-mixes analyzed in this study had a higher sodium content than agreed. We therefore consider it essential to include French bread premixes in the list of sodium reduction products.

The last study published on the sodium content of French bread in Brazil took place in 2015[10] , in which an average of 736 mg/100g of bread was observed and only five samples showed values lower than the maximum established content (616 mg for the year 2012). In this study, the average sodium content of bread produced in the capital of the state of Goiás was well below that of the previous study. Thus, compliance with the voluntary agreement was observed in most of the places studied, with only an average of 2 samples out of the 23 analyzed having a higher content than the agreement, considering a value of 586 mg/100 g of sodium (target for the end of 2014).

However, 78% of the locations reported that they had not changed the recipe, meaning that they could already produce bread with a low sodium content, so it is believed that Goiás must be one of the five states that already had adequate bread in the previous monitoring published by ANVISA .[10]

The variability, although not significant, in the sodium levels between the samples indicates a lack of standardization in the production of French bread, despite reports of the use of technical data sheets and scales and the occurrence of training at most of the sites. Therefore, based on the sodium values observed in this study, a new, more effective reduction is proposed, given that the target suggests gradual reductions over time.

The Brazilian Term of Commitment defined a 10% reduction in sodium in bread over 3 years, i.e. a maximum of 1.44g salt/100g bread by 2014. In European countries such as Italy, in 2009, initial reductions of 15% of salt in bread were proposed by 2011 and further reductions in the following 2 to 3 years[27] . The United Kingdom set an average target of 1 g salt/100 g of bread in 2012 and revised the target to a range of 0.9 g to 1.13 g salt/100 g for 2017 .[28]

It is also worth considering that the Term of Commitment established that from 2015, new targets for the gradual reduction of sodium content in bread should be discussed for the following years, based on tests of new formulations and sensory analyses to detect consumer sensitivity to the reduction in formulations[6] . However, no new reductions have yet been proposed, resulting in a delay of more than two years to the present day. With the recommendation of a further 10% reduction for the following years (reaching 20%), we would reach 1.29 g salt/100 g of bread, which is still well below what is established in other countries.

As for the limitations of this study, it is difficult to obtain the universe of local supermarkets, since the data from the Sanitary Surveillance Department is not available.

Municipal were out of date. There was also a need to explore the frequency of training. Another limitation of the study was that the questionnaire data collection included reported data that was not observed *on site*.

Conclusion

It was observed that the sodium content of the bread analyzed was mostly adequate in relation to the proposed voluntary agreement, which suggests that the target for the state of Goiás was inadequate, as it was based on an overestimated sodium content, based on other products, which is not the reality of the state. The breads had different weights per unit and were much higher than 50g, which could lead to a higher than expected consumption of sodium per portion. As for the production method, the supermarkets that reported changing the salt in the recipe in recent years actually had bread with a lower sodium content than the others. In addition, most of the supermarkets studied manufacture their own bread and these breads had a lower sodium content than those that use bread premix. Therefore, pre-mix manufacturers should reduce the sodium content of their products in order to have a greater impact on the health of the population. It is also suggested that French bread premixes be included in the list of products for sodium reduction in the new targets to be proposed.

The lowest sodium value observed in this study is half the value proposed by the Term of Commitment, which suggests that even greater reductions are possible and can be made without jeopardizing acceptability and without any perceptible change in taste for consumers.

It is believed that voluntary sodium reduction is a good strategy, provided it is well thought out, dealt with on an ongoing basis and monitored to discuss new targets, emphasizing the importance of a greater effort on the part of the government, a greater commitment on the part of industry and health promotion institutions.

REFERENCES

1- Duncan BB, Chor D, Aquino EML, Bensenor IM, Mill JG, Schmidt MI, Lotufo PA, Vigo A, Barreto SM. Chronic non-communicable diseases in Brazil: priority for confrontation and research. Rev Saùde Pùblica. 2012; 46 (suppl. 1):126-134

2- -Malta DC, Neto OLM, Junor JBS. Presentation of the strategic action plan for tackling chronic non-communicable diseases in Brazil, 2011 to 2022 Epidemiol Serv Saùde. 2011 ; 20(4):425-38.

3-Brown I, Tzoulaki I, Candeias V, Elliot P. Salt intake worldwide: implications for public health. Int J Epidemiol. 2009; 38(3):791-813.

4- He FJ, Macgregor GA. A comprehensive review on salt and health and current experience of worldwide salt reduction programs. J Hum Hypertens. 2009; 23(6):363-84.

5- Ministry of Health. Health Surveillance Secretariat, Health Situation Analysis Department. Strategic action plan for tackling chronic non-communicable diseases in Brazil 2011 - 2022. Brasilia: Ministry of Health, 2011.

6- Ministry of Health. Term of Commitment between the Ministry of Health and the Brazilian Food Industry Association (ABIA), the Brazilian Pasta Industry Association (ABIMA), the Brazilian Wheat Industry Association (ABITRIGO) and the Brazilian Bakery and Confectionery Industry Association (ABIP) with the aim of establishing national targets for reducing the sodium content in processed foods in Brazil. Brasilia - DF. 2011

7- Brazilian Institute of Geography and Statistics. Family budget survey 2008-2009: household food purchases per capita: Brazil and Major Regions. Rio de Janeiro: IBGE, 2010.

8- Center for Applied Studies in Nutrition. UNICAMP. TACO - Brazilian Table of Food Composition. 4. ed. Campinas, UNICAMP, 2011.

9- World Health Organization. Guideline: sodium intake for adults and children. Geneva: WHO Library Cataloguing-in-Publication Data; 2012, reprinted 2014.

10-- National Health Surveillance Agency. Ministry of Health (Brazil). Technical report n. 69/2015: sodium content in processed foods. Brasilia, DF: ANVISA, 2015

11- Ferrante D, Apro N, Ferreira V, Virgolini M, Aguilar V, Sosa M., Perel P, Casas J. Feasibility of salt reduction in processed foods in Argentina. Rev Panam Salud Pùblica. 2011; (29) 2:69-75.

12- Brazilian Institute of Geography and Statistics. Micro and small commercial and service companies in Brazil: 2001. IBGE, Coordination of Services and Trade: Rio de Janeiro, 2003.

13- Rosner B. Fundamentals of biostatistics. 7 ed. Brooks/Cole: Cengage Learning, 2011.

14-- Brazil. Resolution RDC No. 359, of December 23, 2003. Technical regulation on portions of packaged foods for nutritional labeling purposes. Diàrio Oficial da Uniâo, Brasilia, DF, 26 dec. 2003.

15- Association of Official Analytical Chemists. Official methods of analysis of the Association of Official Analytical Chemists. Arlington: A.O.A.C., 2011, 18. ed., 4. ed. rev.

16- Adolf Lutz Institute. Physico-chemical methods for food analysis. Sâo Paulo: Instituto Adolfo Lutz, 1. ed. online, 2008.

17- Food Standards Agency. Salt: the facts, United Kingdom, 2012. Accessed on: 2016 Mar 25. Available at: <http://www.nhs.uk/Livewell/ Goodfood/Pages/salt.aspx>

18- Brazil. State Law No. 19289, of May 4, 2016. Official Gazette/GO no. 22319

19- Brazil. Resolution no. 466, of December 12, 2012. Official Journal of the Union, Brasilia, DF, 2013.

20- Ribeiro P, Morais TB, Colugnati FAB, Sigulem DM. Food chemical composition tables: comparative analysis with laboratory results. Rev Saùde Pùblica. 2003; 37(2):216-225.

21- Brazil. Resolution RDC ANVISA/MS no 263, of September 22, 2005. Technical Regulation for cereal products, starches, flours and meals. Official Journal of the Union, Brasilia, DF, September 23, 2005.

22- Pan American Health Organization Nutritional Profile Model. Washington, DC: PAHO, 2016. Accessed on: 2017 Apr 05. Available at: < http://iris.paho.org/xmlui/handle/123456789/18623>.

23- World Health Organization. A comprehensive global monitoring framework including indicators and a set of voluntary global targets for the prevention and control of non-communicable diseases. Accessed on: 2016 Sep 19. Available at:< http://www.who.int/nmh/events/2012/ discussion_paper2_20120322.pdf> .

24- Department of Primary Care, Secretariat of Health Care, Ministry of Health. National Food and Nutrition Policy. Series B. Textos Bàsicos de Saù; 2012

25- Department of Primary Care, Secretariat of Health Care, Ministry of Health. Food guide for the Brazilian population. 2nd Ed. Brasilia: Ministério da Saùde; 2014.

26-- Brandâo SS, Lira HL. Bakery and confectionery technology. Recife: EDUFRPE, 2011. Accessed on: 2017 Apr 05. Available at: < http://www.abip.org.br/site/wp-content/uploads/2016/03/Technologia_de_Panificacao_e_Confeitaria.pdf>.

27-- Strazzullo P, Cairella G, Campanozzi A, Carcea M, Galeone D, Galletti F, Giampaoli S, lacoviello L, Scalfi L. Population based strategy for dietary salt intake reduction: Italian initiatives in the European framework. Nutr Metab Cardiovas Dis. 2012; 22(3):161-6.

28- Food Standards Agency. Salt reduction targets for 2017. United Kingdom, 2014. Accessed on: 2016 Aug 20. Available in: <http://www.food.gov.uk/northern-ireland/nutritionni/salt-ni/salt_targets>

CHAPTER 3 - SCIENTIFIC ARTICLE 2

Title: French bread in Brazil: history, consumption and sodium content

Authors: Thais Braga de Paula[1]

[1] Postgraduate Program in Nutrition and Health, Faculty of Nutrition, Universidade Federal de Goiàs, Goiânia, Goiàs, Brazil.

SUMMARY

In general, bread of all kinds is a staple of the world's diet. In Brazil, French bread occupies a prominent place. Due to its popularity and representativeness in Brazilian eating habits, and because it contains high levels of sodium, it contributes to the maximum daily intake recommended by the World Health Organization. For this reason, there are many studies in the literature suggesting new formulations. Most of them seek improvements in nutritional value by adding ingredients or in acceptability by reducing the sodium content. This paper presents a review of French bread, from its origin and importance in human history to its current habit of consumption, the levels of sodium content and its consequences for the health of the population.

Key words: sodium chloride in the diet, bread, salt, health, eating habits, history.

INTRODUCTION

Bread, according to Resolution RDC No. 263, of September 22, 2005, of Brazil's National Health Surveillance Agency, is the product obtained from wheat flour and/or other flours, with added liquid, resulting from the process of fermentation or not and cooking, and may contain other ingredients, as long as they do not disfigure the products. They can have different toppings, fillings, shapes and textures .[1]

Bread has been one of the most studied food products in terms of its technological properties such as the elasticity of the dough, the appearance of the crust, the crunchiness of the crust, the volume and flavor of the bread in different production situations (dough treatment, wheat quality, among others) .[2]

It is considered a basic component of the Brazilian diet and includes various types such as French bread, the most consumed (58% of bread production), followed by bread rolls, bisnaguinha bread, potato bread, corn bread, hot dog bread, hamburger bread, among others[3] . Other classifications include white bread, wholemeal bread, artisan or rustic bread, black bread and ethnic bread (Pitta, ciabatta, focaccia, baguette, bagel, challat) .[4]

In Brazil, the popularity of bread is due to various factors such as the convenience of being a ready-to-eat product, the many options and different flavors available, its excellent sensory characteristics, the low cost of production (raw materials, machinery and labor) and the fact that it is easily accessible to all age groups and social classes. It can be found in thousands of bakeries and supermarkets, which means that the bakery and confectionery segment in the country now has an annual turnover of US$ 84.7 billion .[5]

Among the breads most consumed by Brazilians is French bread. Data from the National Food Survey (Inquérito Nacional de Alimentaçâo), included in the latest Family Budget Survey (Pesquisa de Orçamentos Familiares - POF) from 2008 to 2009, shows that French bread is the fourth most consumed product among Brazilians, with *per capita* consumption estimated at 53 g *per* day[3] , which is equivalent to one unit *per* day, or approximately one portion .[6]

Due to its importance in eating habits, there are several studies that propose enriching bread with by-products or other functional ingredients. Generally, the main purpose is to provide more nutrients or special components[7-9] . In addition, the partial substitution of wheat flour with another grain or tuber has already been targeted, especially in studies begun in the 1960s, 1970s and 1980s, to reduce the cost of importing wheat into Brazil[10] , which is explored in this article below. Other studies focus on maintaining the quality and acceptability of bread by reducing the sodium content .[11-14]

In view of the above, given the importance of this issue on the world stage for the food industry and public health, the aim of this study was to carry out a review of French bread, from its origin and importance in human history to the present day, when it has become a daily habit of consumption, relating the levels of sodium content and its consequences for the health of the population.

METHODS

A review was carried out using the Scielo, Food Science Technology Abstracts (FSTA) and Medline databases. Key words used in the bibliographic search were: bread, sodium chloride, salt, history of bread and technology. Economic data from bakery associations, statistical data and surveys from the Brazilian Institute of Geography and Statistics, as well as legislation in force in Brazil on the subject, were added to the articles selected. The search was carried out for works from the 1980s onwards, due to the historical data, and the aim was to give greater emphasis to works published in the last 15 years, the period in which the proposed theme acquired greater relevance in the scientific environment.

BREAD HISTORY

The development of bread (the baking of a dough made with flour from certain cereals, wheat being the most widely accepted, water and salt) is closely linked to the history of humanity, from the first loaf of bread to the present day. For the people who eat it, bread has cultural, economic, political, religious and even artistic meanings .[15]

The use of bread in food originated thousands of years before Christ. Initially, different grains were crushed between stones to obtain a flour that was added to soups and porridges. Later, other ingredients were added to the flour, such as honey, sweet olive oil, grape must, eggs and ground meat, forming a kind of cake that was baked on hot stones or under ashes. This type of cake was considered a food that preceded bread itself .[15]

Historical data, such as cave paintings from 3000 to 4000 years BC, show the Egyptians as the possible discoverers of the process of fermenting wheat, the basis for making bread, in order to make the dough lighter and softer. The Egyptians were also the first to use clay ovens, replacing the process of baking on hot stones or under ashes .[8]

Over time, man improved his bread-making techniques, introducing fermentation alongside baking. One of man's main activities during the classical Greco-Roman period was the act of producing bread, which led to an increase in the number of public bakeries during the period .[16]

Population growth from the tenth to the end of the thirteenth century led to a huge expansion in wheat cultivation and by the end of the fourteenth century, Italian city dwellers were baking bread almost exclusively with wheat flour .[17]

It is worth adding that the expansion of new flour milling processes contributed greatly to the bakery industry. Wheat grains, previously ground in manual stone mills, moved on to stone mills powered by animals, then by water, wind and finally steam .[15]

With the Industrial Revolution, various new products were developed due to the mechanization that was increasingly common among bakeries. Some breads became typical of the region or country in which they were produced, such as black bread in Russia and French bread in France , .[516]

In Brazil, there are reports that French bread began to be made at the end of the 19th century. At this time, people began to switch from eating a type of bread with a dark crust and crumb, made from corn or cassava flour, to a bread recipe brought over by European immigrants made from wheat flour, with a golden crust and crumb .[16]

In the 20th century, the quality of French-style bread in Brazil evolved along with the expansion of French-style bakeries and patisseries, a culture that was influential in the country at the time. It also began to use mainly male labor, replacing female labor, which at the time dominated the entire bread-making process[18] . Since then, French bread has become part of Brazilian eating habits .[5]

SODIUM CONSUMPTION AND REDUCTION STRATEGIES IN BAKERY PRODUCTS

In recent decades, salt consumption in most countries has been excessive, ranging from 9 to 12 g per person per day[19] . The World Health Organization (WHO) recommends a daily intake for adults of no more than 5 g of salt (2000 mg of sodium)[20] . Evidence also suggests that sodium intake should be even lower, from 1200 to 1500 mg/day, considering its impact on health[21] . In Brazil, about 4.7 g/day of sodium is consumed, which totals almost 12 g/day of salt .[22]

The well-established relationship between high sodium intake and the onset of chronic non-communicable diseases, including cardiovascular diseases such as hypertension, myocardial infarction and stroke[2] 3,2[4] , is one of the reasons for reducing the daily recommendations for this nutrient.

Studies also point to the positive correlation between its intake and some diseases such as gastric cancer[21] , kidney stones[22] , diabetes, osteoporosis, reduced bone density, alongside other factors such as obesity, smoking and a sedentary lifestyle .[19,27]

The scientific evidence regarding sodium intake and blood pressure elevation has been pointed out as one of the strongest cause and effect relationships among all existing dietary factors associated with the onset of cardiovascular diseases, which justifies global initiatives to reduce consumption of this nutrient .[28,29]

In the midst of this, the Ministry of Health has set a target in the National Health Plan 2012-2015 of reducing sodium consumption by 25%, from 12g to 9g by 2015. To try to reach this target, measures are being taken to raise awareness among the population and agreements are being reached between the government and representatives of the food industry .[30]

Among the agreements signed is a commitment agreement between the Ministry of Health and the Brazilian Food Industry Association (ABIA), the Brazilian Pasta Industry Association (ABIMA), the Brazilian Wheat Industry Association (ABITRIGO) and the Brazilian Bakery and Confectionery Industry Association (ABIP) to reduce the sodium content in baked goods. Breads were selected as a priority area for actions to reduce salt and sodium .[31]

This selection was based on the data revealed in various technical reports carried out by ANVISA[32-35] . In 2012[34] , the average sodium content found for bread in general was 368 mg/100g of bread and for bread rolls 475 mg/100g. The following year[35] , the loaves of bread analyzed had average values of more than 499 mg/100g and the bisnaguinha type loaves had average levels of 470 mg/100g of bread.

This Term of Commitment stipulated that biscuits, bread rolls and French rolls should have a gradual 10% reduction in sodium content, from 2% to 1.8% of this mineral for every 100 grams of wheat flour. The reduction should take place from 2011 to 201436.

CHALLENGES IN REDUCING SALT IN BREAD

There are challenges to reducing salt in food. The main ones concern technological aspects and acceptability.

In the bakery industry in particular, salt stands out for firming up the gluten network and making it more stable and less extensible. It also helps with the fermentation process, because the more salt you add to the dough, the longer the yeast has to act. With this longer time, more gas is released, thus increasing the expansion of the bread and improving the texture, making it softer .[37]

Alternatives to these important functions of salt for the final product are being studied in order to bring new formulations without losses in terms of texture, palatability and visual appearance.

One of the aspects studied is the partial and gradual replacement of sodium chloride with potassium chloride in the French bread recipe. The negative characteristics of potassium chloride are its high cost and its bitter and astringent aftertaste, which affects the final taste of the product and prevents it from being used frequently. However, its positive characteristics include the benefits caused by potassium ions for the cardiovascular health of individuals, as well as the reduction of sodium and its excess consequences for health[3] 8. The combined use of potassium chloride and sodium chloride (0.6% and 1.4% respectively of the total mass of bread) in the manufacture of French bread did not drastically affect the final product in attributes such as appearance, aroma and taste .[39]

Other substitutes for sodium chloride are possible and should be studied, including monosodium glutamate (MSG), other additives and even the use of wholemeal flours.

MSG is the sodium salt of glutamic acid, considered a flavor enhancer and one of the factors responsible for the umami flavor[40] . Although the structure of MSG contains sodium, it is known that the sodium content is much lower than that of table salt (the equivalent of 123 mg of Na/1g of MSG and 400 mg of sodium/100g of NaCL, respectively).

The use of an inhomogeneous sodium distribution strategy, without the use of sodium substitutes, flavor or aroma additives, increased the intensity of the salty taste by up to 117% in the bread dough and proved to be effective in reducing salt for the manufacture of baked goods[41] . This increase in intensity was due to the contrast of flavors in the bread dough, and it was possible to reduce the salt content of the preparation by up to 28% without reducing the perception of the usual salt. However, the acceptability of these products has only been verified on a laboratory scale and has not yet been tested with consumers.

Breads made with 50% whole wheat flour and a 10% reduction in sodium were not perceived by North American consumers. Although a 30% reduction in sodium was detected, it did not bring any negative aspects to the evaluation[12] , which also occurred with Dutch university student consumers when they analyzed the acceptability of wholemeal breads with a 52% reduction in sodium content and a variety of fillings[1] 4. The progressive and gradual reduction of the sodium content in white bread by up to 25% over six weeks did not influence the acceptability of Australian consumers .[13]

It is known that formulating a French bread without salt is still a difficult task. The taste buds of Brazilian consumers are used to eating foods with high levels of salt, and French bread without added salt and without gradual adaptation to its reduction ends up tasting sweeter, which is different from the characteristic and well-accepted taste of this type of bread. Changes have been made to the formulation to reduce the sweet taste, but they leave a neutral or tasteless flavor in the bread .[11]

Unpublished data from the authors of this review showed that the sodium content of French bread made in supermarket bakeries in Goiânia-GO, analyzed in the laboratory, ranged from 286 to 702 mg/100 g of bread (corresponding to 0.72 g and 1.76 g of salt). Only two supermarkets obtained bread samples above 586 mg, the maximum reference value in the Term of Commitment. Samples were taken from 23 medium-sized and large supermarkets and a questionnaire was administered in the places visited to find out about aspects related to the way bread is produced. They observed that the supermarkets that use their own recipe make bread with a lower sodium content than those that use a pre-mix, basically wheat flour and salt, ready for making the bread. They also observed that the majority of the sites studied were in line with the voluntary agreement between the Ministry of Health and the bakery industries, presenting bread with a reduced sodium content, with no difference between the samples taken. However, as 78% of the sites reported that they had not changed their recipe in recent years, the sites could already be producing bread with a low sodium content. Therefore, for further reductions, the sodium values defined as the maximum limit should be reviewed.

Thus, based on what has been observed in the literature, it can be concluded that more longitudinal studies are needed to verify, in different populations, what minimum salt content is necessary to make French bread that is well accepted by consumers and whose reductions are really effective for the health of the population.

COMMENTS AND CONCLUSIONS

Bread has been a much-studied food in the literature and for this reason, studies with new formulations have gained relevance in the scientific world. In most cases, new formulations of bread have better nutritional quality and, due to their widespread consumption and popularity, can bring more health benefits to consumers.

It is known that there are many types of bread and that each one has its own sensory and nutritional characteristics. French bread was chosen for this review because of its popularity in Brazil. It is important to look at bread beyond salt, as it is still an accessible and interesting choice for a large part of the population. People with a higher risk of cardiovascular disease should pay attention to all the foods they eat during the day, avoiding more than one portion of those with a high sodium content. In addition, when eating French bread, they should pay attention to the fillings they choose, which are usually high in sodium, such as cheese, salted margarine and sausages in general.

This highlights the need to continue with public policies aimed at gradually reducing the amount of salt in French bread, so that one unit of bread contributes much less to an individual's daily sodium requirement.

Sources of funding: Master's degree scholarship/CAPES awarded to Paula,

T.B., Young Talents Scholarship/CNPQ awarded to Alexandre da Silva Soares.

The authors declare no conflict of interest.

Acknowledgments: The authors would like to thank the Coordination of Improvement of Higher Education Personnel (CAPES) for granting a master's degree scholarship.

REFERENCES

1- Brazil. Resolution RDC ANVISA/MS no. 263, of September 22, 2005. Technical regulation for cereal products, starches, flours and meals. Official Journal of the Union, Brasilia, DF, September 23, 2005.

2- Baardseth P, Kvaal, K, Lea P, Ellenkjaer MR, Faergestad EM. The Effects of the Bread Making Process and Wheat Quality on French Baguettes. J Cereal Sci. 2000; 32:73-87.

3- Brazilian Institute of Geography and Statistics - IBGE. Pesquisa de orçamentos familiares 2008-2009: aquisição alimentar domiciliar per capita: Brasil e Grandes Regiões. 2010 [Accessed 2015 Feb 25]. Available at: http://www.ibge.gov.br/home/estatistica/populacao

/condicaodevida/pof/2008_2009_aquisicao/pof20082009_aquisicao.pdf.

4- - Canella-Rawls S. Bread - Art and Science. Sâo Paulo: Editora Senac, 2005.

5- Brazilian Association of Bakery and Confectionery Industries - ABIP. About the sector 2015 and History of bread. [Accessed 2016 Jun 07]. Available at: http://www.abip.org.br/site/sobre-o-setor-2015/.

6- - Brazil. Resolution RDC No. 359, of December 23, 2003. Technical regulation on portions of packaged foods for nutritional labeling purposes. Diàrio Oficial da Uniâo, Brasilia, DF, 26 dec. 2003.

7-El-Soukkary FAH. Evaluation of pumpkin seed products for bread fortification. Plant Foods Hum Nutr. 2001; 56:365-384.

8- Bowles S, Demiate IM. Physico-chemical characterization of okara and its application in French bread. Cienc Tecnol Aliment. 2006;26(3):652-659.

9- Souto, TS, Brasil ALD, Taddei JAAC. Acceptability of bread fortified with microencapsulated iron by children from daycare centers in the southern and eastern regions of the city of São Paulo. Rev Nutr. 2008;21(6):647-657.

10-- Brazilian Association of Cassava Starch Producers - ABAM. Our daily bread with cassava! [Accessed 2016 Sep 15]. Available at: http://www.abam.com.br/revista/ revista11/paonossodecadadia.php.

11- -Silva MEMP, Yonamine GH, Mitsuiki L. Development and Evaluation of Homemade Unsalted French Bread. Brazilian J Food Technol. 2003; 6(Suppl.2):229-36.

12- La Croix KW, Fiala SC, Colonna AE, Durham CA, Morrisey MT, Drum DK, et al. Consumer detection and acceptability of reduced-sodium bread. Public Health Nutr. 2015;18(8):1412-1418.

13-- Girgis S, Neal B, Prescott J, Dumbrell S, Turner C, Woodward M. A one-quarter reduction in the salt content of bread can be made without detection. Eur J Clin Nutr. 2003; 57(4):616-620.

14-- Bolhuis DP, Temme EHM, Koeman FT, Noort MWJ, Kremer S, Janssen AM. A salt reduction of 50% in bread does not decrease bread consumption or increase sodium intake by the choice of sandwich fillings. J Nutr. 2011;141(12):2249-2255.

15-- BNDES Sector. Wheat production chain 2003. [Accessed 2017 Mar 05]. Available at:

https://web.bndes.gov.br/bib/jspui/bitstream/1408/2584/1/BS%2018%20Cade i a%20produtiva%20do%20trigo_P.pdf.

16- Bona S. Feasibility studies on the production of French bread from frozen dough. Master's dissertation in Food Engineering. Florianópolis SC, 2002.

17-- Flandin JL, Montanari M. História da Alimentaçâo, 2 ed. Sâo Paulo: Estaçâo Liberdade, 1998.

18- Matos MIS. Portuguese and political experiences: the struggle and the bread: São Paulo 1870-1945. História. 2009;28(Suppl.1):415-43.

19--Brown I, Tzoulaki I, Candeias V, Elliot P. Salt intake worldwide: implications for public health. Int J Epidemiol. 2009; 38(3):791-813.

20- World Health Organization. Guideline: Sodium intake for adults and children. Geneva: WHO; 2012.

21- Dotsh M, Busch J, Batenburg M, Liem G, Tareilus E, Mueller R, Meijer G. Strategies to reduce sodium consumption: a food industry perspective. Crit Rev Food Sci Nutr. 2009; 49:841-851.

22- Sarno F, Claro RM, Levy RB, Bandoni DH, Monteiro CA. Estimated sodium intake by the Brazilian population, 2008-2009. Rev Saude Publica. 2013;47(Suppl.3):571-578.

23- O'Donnell MJ, Yusuf S, Mente A, Gao P, Mann JF, Teo K, McQueen M, et al. Urinary sodium and potassium excretion and risk of cardiovascular events. N Engl J Med. 2011; 371:612-623.

24- Theodore AK, Cowley AW, Frohlich, ED. Salt in health and disease - a delicate balance. N Engl J Med. 2013;368(13):1229-1237.

25-- Tsugane S, Sasazuki S, Kobayashi M, Sasaki, S. Salt and salted food intake and subsequent risk of gastric cancer among middle-aged Japanese men and women. Br J Cancer. 2004; 90(1):128-134.

26- Obligado SH, Goldfarb, DS. The association of nephrolithiasis with hypertension and obesity: a review. Am J Hypertens. 2008; 21(3):257-264.

27- He FJ, Macgregor GA. A comprehensive review on salt and health and current experience of worldwide salt reduction programs. J Hum Hypertens.

2009; 23(6):363-384.

28- Kotchen TA, Cowley AW, Frohlic ED. Salt in health and disease: a delicate balance. N Engl J Med. 2013; 368(13):1229-1237.

29- World Health Organization - WHO. Reducing salt intake in populations. Report of a WHO Forum and Technical Meeting, 5-7 October 2006, Paris, France. [Accessed2015 Jan12]. Availableat :

http://www.who.int/dietphysicalactivity/reducingsaltintake_EN.pdf.

30--Nilson EAF, Jaime PC, Resende DO. Initiatives developed in Brazil to reduce the sodium content of processed foods. Rev Panam Salud Pùblica. 2012; 32(Suppl.4):287-92.

31- - Ministry of Health. Term of Commitment between the Ministry of Health and the Brazilian Food Industry Association (ABIA), the Brazilian Pasta Industry Association (ABIMA), the Brazilian Wheat Industry Association (ABITRIGO) and the Brazilian Bakery and Confectionery Industry Association (ABIP) with the aim of establishing national targets for reducing the sodium content in processed foods in Brazil. Brasilia - DF. 2011.

32-- National Health Surveillance Agency - ANVISA. Ministry of Health (Brazil). Technical report no 43/2010: Nutritional profile of processed foods. Brasilia, DF: ANVISA, 2010. 52 p. [Accessed 2015 Mar 23]. Available em: http://portal.anvisa.gov.br/wps/wcm/connect/c476ee0047457a6e86efd63fbc4c6735/INFORME+T%C3%89CNICO+n++43+-+2010-

+PERFIL+NUTRICIONAL+_2_.pdf ?MOD=AJPERES.

33- National Health Surveillance Agency - ANVISA. Ministry of Health (Brazil). Technical report no. *502012:* Sodium content of processed foods. Brasilia, DF: ANVISA, 2012b. 27 p. [Accessed 2015 Mar 23]. Available at: http: //www.nutritotal.com.br/diretrizes/files/271-INFORME_TECNICO Anvisa_Processed.pdf

- National Health Surveillance Agency. Ministry of Health (Brazil). Technical report no. 542013: Sodium content of processed foods. Brasilia, DF: ANVISA, 2013.21 p. [Accessed 2015 Mar 23]. Available in:http://portal.anvisa.gov.br/ wps/wcm/connect/8ab9538040695edd83fed3dc5a12ff52/INFORME+T%C3% 89CNICO+JULHO+2013.pdf?MOD=AJPERES.

34- National Health Surveillance Agency. Ministry of Health (Brazil) Technical Report No. 61/2014: Sodium content in processed foods. Brasilia, DF: ANVISA, 2014. [Accessed 2015 Mar 23]. Available at: http://s.anvisa.gov.br/wps/wcm/connect/1e d11a004512fdc681bdf9e784b81089/INFORME+T%C3%89CNICO+N.+61+A GOSTO+2014.pdf?MOD=AJPERES.

35- - Brazilian Institute for Consumer Protection. Sodium reduction in food: An analysis of voluntary agreements in Brazil, Sâo Paulo, 2014. Sâo Paulo: IDEC; 2014. (Idec Notebooks - Food Series).

36- - Hutton T. Sodium Technological functions of salt in the manufacturing of food and drink products. Br Food J. 2002; 104(2):126-152.

37- Du C, Zhang Y, El H A, Dempesey CE, Hancox JC. Ranolazine inhibition of hERG potassium channels: drug-pore interaction and reduced potency aganst inactivation mutants. J Mol Cell Cardiol. 2014;74:220-230.

38- Ignàcio AKF, Rodrigues JTD, Niizu PY, Chang YK, Stell CJ. Effect of replacing sodium chloride with potassium chloride in French bread. Brazilian J Food Technol 2013;16(Suppl.1):01-11.

39- Jinap S, Hajeb P. Glutamate. Its applications in food and contribution to health. Appetite 2010; 55(Suppl.1):1-10.

40--Noort MWJ, Bult JHF, Stieger M, Hamer RJ. Saltiness enhancement in bread by inhomogeneous spatial distribution of sodium chloride. Journal of Cereal Science. 2010; 52: 378-386.

FINAL CONSIDERATIONS

The proposal for this work arose from an invitation to take part in a Working Group set up by the Legislative Assembly. The "Working Group for the Reduction of Sodium, Sugars and Fats in Food in the State of Goiás" is made up of different social actors, from various professions and positions, which in addition to its heterogeneity, brings social representation. For this reason, since there was a need to study issues involved with the group, we decided to work with sodium in a product that is highly consumed by the Brazilian population and which has not yet been studied much: French bread.

So, as a first idea, we planned to study bread produced in bakeries in general in Goiânia-GO, but data on the universe of bakeries for sample calculation was out of date, which led to the choice of studying supermarket bakeries that had a smaller universe and were easier to obtain and/or check.

In addition, it was important to take a scientific stance in order to verify all the information provided by representatives of the group, given that we were told that all the French bread manufacturers were already compliant and that the vast majority used bread premix in their production, which was also already compliant, according to studies that were not presented to us. Fortunately, we decided to continue with the study and found that the reality didn't quite match the reports.

Another interesting factor during the study was working with a scholarship holder from the Young Talents Program/CNPQ, who helped in the development of the analyses, including a co-supervision experience.

In relation to the results, most of the French bread samples analyzed were adequate in relation to what was proposed in the Term of Commitment between the Ministry of Health and the industries, and it is possible that in some bakeries the sodium content had already been reduced due to the report of no changes in the ingredients of the recipes over the last four years.

The lowest sodium value observed in this study is half the value proposed by the Term of Commitment, which suggests that even greater reductions are possible and can be made without jeopardizing acceptability and without altering consumers' perceptions of taste.

In addition, most of the supermarkets studied produce their own bread and this bread had a lower sodium content compared to the places that use pre-mixed bread. Therefore, pre-mix manufacturers should reduce the sodium content of their products in order to have a greater impact on the health of the population. It is also suggested that French bread premixes be included in the list of products for sodium reduction in the new targets that will be proposed.

Therefore, considering that in Brazil there are still other products besides French bread on the voluntary salt reduction list, this strategy could be rethought in order to better understand the current sodium content of foods, i.e. the real sodium content, in order to propose a significant reduction that could bring more convincing results.

A voluntary agreement reduction must be dealt with continuously and monitored in order to discuss new targets. With regard to French bread, there is a delay of two years and a few months in evaluating and continuing new reductions, highlighting the need for greater effort on the part of the government, a greater commitment on the part of industry and health promotion institutions.

APPENDICES

APPENDIX A - Questionnaire

1- Trade name and company name of the establishment:

2- Size: ( ) Medium ( ) Large

3- Address, telephone number and e-mail address of the establishment:

4- How is your French bread made?

( ) I make my own French bread from the ingredients (e.g. wheat flour, yeast, water...)

( ) I make bread from French bread pre-mix

5- What is the average number of French breads made per day (in kg)?

6- Does the preparation of French bread have a technical sheet?

( ) Yes ( ) No

7- Is the technical data sheet used in the manufacturing process?

( ) Yes, it is used by all bakers

( ) It is used by some of the bakers, but not all of them

( ) Not used by any baker

( ) Not applicable (those without a technical file)

8- Do you use scales when making French bread? *

( ) Yes ( ) No

9- If so, how accurate is the scale (1 in 1g, 2 in 2g, 5 in 5g)?

10- Employees involved in the manufacturing process receive any kind of training for standardized bread making?

( ) Yes ( ) No

11- How long have you been using the current recipe?

12- Has there been any change in the quantity of any of the ingredients in the current recipe?

( ) Yes

( ) No

( ) I can't answer

If so, which ingredient? ______________________

APPENDIX B - TCLE

INFORMED CONSENT FORM - TCLE

You are being invited to take part, as a volunteer, in the research entitled "Salt and sodium in bakery products". My name is Thais Braga de Paula, I am the researcher in charge and my area of expertise is nutrition. After receiving the following clarifications and information, if you agree to take part in the study, please sign at the end of this document, which is printed in two copies, one of which is yours and the other belongs to the researcher in charge. I would like to make it clear that if you refuse to take part, you will not be penalized in any way. However, if you agree to take part, the researcher(s) in charge will be able to answer any questions you may have about the research via e-mail (thaisbpaula@hotmail.com) and even by calling collect on the following telephone number(s): (62) 982694947. If you still have any doubts *about your rights* as a participant in this research, you can also contact the **Research Ethics Committee of** the Federal University of Goiás, on (62)3521-1215.

1. Important information about the research:

The title of this work is 'Salt and sodium in bakery products' and the importance of this study is to help monitor the sodium content in the state of Goiás, compliance with the voluntary agreement "Sodium Reduction Plan for Processed Foods", signed by food industries and the Ministry of Health. The aim of the study was to analyze the sodium content and production/marketing methods of French bread produced in supermarket bakeries in the municipality of Goiânia-GO.

Your participation only consists of answering a simple questionnaire about bread-making in your workplace. The interview will not be recorded or filmed. It is also worth remembering that your participation does not involve any discomfort or physical or psychosocial risk and helps us to trace the way in which French bread is produced in the city of Goiânia.

Your participation in the survey does not involve any kind of payment or financial reward, nor does it involve any expenses to the participant. We guarantee the privacy of your data and the name of the company will not be disclosed. You are free to refuse to take part in the survey by answering the questionnaire or withdrawing your consent, without any penalty.

1.1 Consent for the Participation of the Person as a Research Subject:

Me, ,

registered under RG/CPF ...., undersigned,

I agree to take part in the study entitled "Salt and sodium content in bakery products". I inform you that I am over 18 years of age and that my participation in this study is voluntary. I have also been duly informed by the researcher in charge, Tânia Aparecida Pinto de Castro Ferreira, about the research, the procedures and methods involved, as well as the possible risks and benefits arising from my participation in the study. I have been assured that I can withdraw my consent at any time, without this leading to any penalty. I therefore declare that I agree to take part in the research project described above.

Goiânia, ... from .... of ....

Full signature of participant

Full signature of the researcher responsible

FACULTY OF NUTRITION - FANUT/UFG

Rua 227 Qd. 68 s/n° - Setor Leste Universitàrio - Goiânia - Goiàs - Brazil - CEP: 74.605-080

(62) 3209-6270

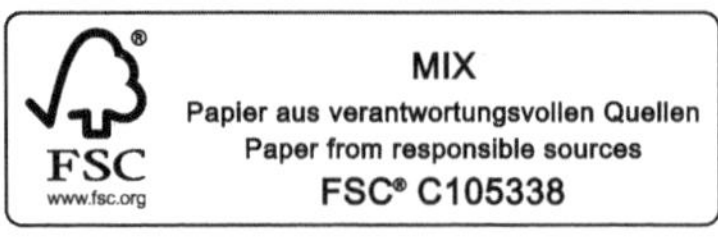

Printed by Books on Demand GmbH, Norderstedt / Germany